D1795861

EYE AND VISION RESEARCH DEVELOPMENTS

ALLERGIC DISORDERS
OF THE OCULAR SURFACE

EYE AND VISION RESEARCH DEVELOPMENTS

Additional books in this series can be found on Nova's website
under the Series tab.

Additional e-books in this series can be found on Nova's website
under the e-book tab.

ALLERGIES AND INFECTIOUS DISEASES

Additional books in this series can be found on Nova's website
under the Series tab.

Additional e-books in this series can be found on Nova's website
under the e-book tab.

EYE AND VISION RESEARCH DEVELOPMENTS

ALLERGIC DISORDERS
OF THE OCULAR SURFACE

DE GAULLE I. CHIGBU

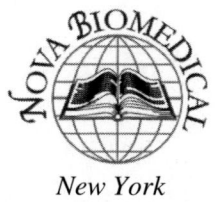

New York

Copyright © 2013 by Nova Science Publishers, Inc.

All rights reserved. No part of this book may be reproduced, stored in a retrieval system or transmitted in any form or by any means: electronic, electrostatic, magnetic, tape, mechanical photocopying, recording or otherwise without the written permission of the Publisher.

For permission to use material from this book please contact us:
Telephone 631-231-7269; Fax 631-231-8175
Web Site: http://www.novapublishers.com

NOTICE TO THE READER

The Publisher has taken reasonable care in the preparation of this book, but makes no expressed or implied warranty of any kind and assumes no responsibility for any errors or omissions. No liability is assumed for incidental or consequential damages in connection with or arising out of information contained in this book. The Publisher shall not be liable for any special, consequential, or exemplary damages resulting, in whole or in part, from the readers' use of, or reliance upon, this material. Any parts of this book based on government reports are so indicated and copyright is claimed for those parts to the extent applicable to compilations of such works.

Independent verification should be sought for any data, advice or recommendations contained in this book. In addition, no responsibility is assumed by the publisher for any injury and/or damage to persons or property arising from any methods, products, instructions, ideas or otherwise contained in this publication.

This publication is designed to provide accurate and authoritative information with regard to the subject matter covered herein. It is sold with the clear understanding that the Publisher is not engaged in rendering legal or any other professional services. If legal or any other expert assistance is required, the services of a competent person should be sought. FROM A DECLARATION OF PARTICIPANTS JOINTLY ADOPTED BY A COMMITTEE OF THE AMERICAN BAR ASSOCIATION AND A COMMITTEE OF PUBLISHERS.

Additional color graphics may be available in the e-book version of this book.

Library of Congress Cataloging-in-Publication Data

ISBN: 978-1-62417-614-2

Library of Congress Control Number: 2012955260

Published by Nova Science Publishers, Inc. † New York

Dedicated to my family for their affection and encouragement
Eziaha, Chidubem, Ekenedirijah

In special memory of my parents for their inspiration
Enyimmiri and Egowure

With special appreciation for the resolute support that made this
accomplishment possible
Prof. Maria Stokes

Contents

Foreword

It is with great honor I write this foreword for De Gaulle I. Chigbu, O.D., M.S. He is a friend and colleague who has dedicated the majority of his career to the study of ocular allergy and its consequences on the human eye. I hate long forewords; in fact, when I open a new book, I usually scan it to see if there is anything interesting. I am sure you will do the same, so let me be short-winded. This book, Allergic Disorders of the Ocular Surface, represents the culmination of years of work and study in an effort to reach out to all ophthalmic colleagues on a commonly presenting and evolving clinical issue.

The book is logically sequenced; opening with a general overview of the subject matter in chapter 1. The second chapter discusses the cells and mediators that play a vital role in the pathomechanism of allergic eye diseases. The third chapter reviews the immunology that is relevant to ocular allergy with emphasis on IgE- and T-lymphocyte mediated hypersensitivity reactions in allergic disorders of the ocular surface and the lymphocyte activation process. The pharmacotherapy of ocular allergy is addressed in chapter 4 with emphasis on the clinical pharmacology of anti-allergic and anti-inflammatory pharmaceutical agents. Chapters 5 – 9 concentrate on specific types of allergic ocular surface diseases. Each chapter is organized into sections that describe the pathomechanism, clinical presentation, the hallmark features necessary for diagnosis, the strategy of management, and the potential complications, which may arise during the management and the general prognosis and expectations given timely treatment.

This book is extraordinarily well-referenced and up to date and complete. I have enjoyed reading it. For those who are interested in the cellular and molecular mechanisms...I assure you it is in here. For those of us who just want some clinical advice....well, that is in here too. Please enjoy this marvelous book, and make use of it to serve your patients. Your use of this textbook to effect positive change in the world is the greatest compliment the author could receive.

Andrew S. Gurwood, O.D.
Professor,
Salus University, Elkins Park, Pennsylvania, US

Preface

An allergic disorder of the ocular surface affects more than 20% of the general population. Allergic eye diseases are those conditions in which IgE-and/or T-lymphocyte mediated mechanisms are involved. They can have a significant impact on an individual's quality of life. Mast cells, eosinophils and CD4$^+$T-lymphocytes, as well as epithelial cells and fibroblasts of the conjunctiva and cornea play a role in the inflammatory process of ocular allergy.

The management of allergic disorders of the ocular surface is aimed at preventing the release of mediators of allergy, controlling the allergic inflammatory cascade and preventing ocular surface damage secondary to the allergic response.

To achieve success in the management of ocular allergy, the clinician requires considerable understanding of the pathomechanisms and clinical features of the different forms of ocular allergy, in addition to adequate knowledge of the treatment modalities. This book addresses these important aspects of allergic disorders of the ocular surface with particular emphasis on the pathomechanism and pharmacotherapy of the different types of ocular allergy.

Thus, the goal of this book is to provide the student and practitioner in eyecare with considerable insight into the pathomechanism and pharmacotherapy of allergic disorders of the ocular surface.

The book is organized into chapters that focus on the different aspects of allergic eye disease and then on specific eye disorders, as outlined by Professor Gurwood in the Foreword. Ocular immunology is a rapidly changing field of ocular medicine and, as such, there are always going to be changes that will affect the clinical care we provide to our patients.

This book will equip you with the basic knowledge for understanding the pathomechanism of allergic eye diseases, as well as the emerging evidence on patient management in this field to help you make informed choices in patient care.

De Gaulle I. Chigbu, O.D., M.S.
Associate Professor
Pennsylvania College of Optometry at Salus University
Elkins Park, Pennsylvania, US

Acknowledgment

I wish to thank a few individuals out of the many who were involved in educating and training me - Drs. Bernadita S. Mencias, Quintus Ngumah, Dominic Onwukwe, Frank Metzstein, Francis Iwuagwu, Ebele Uzodike, Okechi Amaechi, Neal Nyman, and Prof. Roger Buckley.

I would like to thank Drs. Paulinus Chigbu, Shanthy Sandrasekaramudaly-Brown, Jonathan Stevens, Susan Oleszewski, Michelle Hennelly, Bernard Blaustein, Anthony Di Stefano, Thomas Lewis, Jeffrey Nyman, Kelly Malloy, Tiffenie Harris, Aviazu Anomah, Melissa Trego, Ruth Shoge, Chris Rinehart, Richard Bennett, Brandy Scombordi, and Olta Cuci for their help and support over the years. I also recognize the staff and students at Fight for Sight Eye Clinic (London) and The Eye Institute (Philadelphia) for their years of professional support.

Many individuals have provided assistance with other tasks during the course of writing this book. In particular, I would like to thank Nova Science Publishers, Daniel Eke, Sharon Kelly, Marian Weber, Nathalie Campbell, and Luminata Vulca.

The strong mentorship provided by Profs. Polycarp Chigbu and Linda Casser is deeply appreciated.

Finally, for their love, understanding and patience during the time I was writing this book, a special thank you to my wife, Eziaha Chigbu and my children, Chidubem and Ekenedirijah.

Chapter 1

Introduction

Allergy is an over-reaction of the body's immune system to harmless foreign substances or allergens, such as airborne pollen, animal dander, house dust mite, that the body perceives as undesirable. Allergic eye diseases affect more than 20% of the general population [1-3]. Although the incidence of ocular allergy may vary by geographical location, it is more prevalent in individuals that suffer from allergic disorders such as atopic dermatitis and asthma [4]. Ocular allergy ranges in severity from mild forms, which can interfere significantly with one's quality of life, to severe cases with increased potential for causing visual impairment [5].

Allergic disorders of the ocular surface includes perennial allergic conjunctivitis (PAC), seasonal allergic conjunctivitis (SAC), giant papillary conjunctivitis (GPC), vernal keratoconjunctivitis (VKC), atopic keratoconjunctivitis (AKC), and contact ocular allergy (COA) [6]. Seasonal allergens include tree pollen (early spring), grass pollen (May-July), weed (ragweed) pollen (August-October) and outdoor molds such as Cladosporium, Alternaria, epicoccum, aerospora, and basidiospores [7]. The perennial allergens include house dust mites (Dermatophagoides farinea and D. pteronyssinus), indoor molds (aspergillus species (A. flavis and A. fumigates) and penicillium species), feather, cockroaches, and animal dander (dog and cat dander) [7]. Allergic eye conditions have a significant impact on the quality of life and wellbeing of the individual. It can affect learning performance in school-aged individuals and work productivity in adults. Furthermore, it imposes a significant burden on the economy of countries in the form of rising healthcare costs and reduced productivity through lost workdays [8].

Allergic eye disease, an abnormal immune hypersensitivity response to allergens, is predominantly an IgE-mediated and/or T-lymphocyte-mediated immune hypersensitivity reaction that leads to an immune response, resulting in the clinical manifestations of ocular allergy [9]. The key cellular components of ocular allergy are mast cells, eosinophils and T-lymphocytes [4]. Additionally, epithelial cells and fibroblast of the conjunctiva and cornea also play a role in the inflammatory process of ocular allergy [10]. The pathomechanism of acute ocular allergy involves acute antibody (IgE)-mediated mast cell degranulation and minimal presence of migratory inflammatory cells. In chronic ocular allergy, the pathophysiology consists of persistent activation of mast cells and eosinophil-T-lymphocyte-mediated delayed-type hypersensitivity (DTH) response [11-14].

The ocular surface and its adnexa are comprised of the cornea, conjunctiva, the main lacrimal gland, glands of the eyelids, accessory lacrimal glands and the nasolacrimal system [15]. This book will focus on the conjunctiva and cornea, the two major components of the ocular surface affected by allergic inflammatory disorders. Although the conjunctiva is an immunologically active mucosal site, there are several immunoregulatory mechanisms in place to control the innate and adaptive immune response in order to prevent or limit ocular tissue damage [16].

In allergic disorders of the ocular surface, the ocular allergic response usually results from the exposure of allergen-specific IgE on the ocular surface to environmental allergens, which culminates in allergen-induced cross linking of the IgE receptors on the surface of the conjunctival mast cells [6]. This triggers mast cell activation and subsequent release of pro-allergic and pro-inflammatory mediators [6, 17]. The release of these mediators triggers the clinical manifestations of ocular allergy.

Most individuals with ocular allergy present with complaints of itchy, red watery eyes, and may display accompanying conjunctival chemosis and eyelid edema. Skin prick testing or the radioallergosorbent (RAST) test can be used to confirm the diagnosis of allergy and identify the offending allergen [4]. However, skin prick test or RAST are of limited use in diagnosing chronic ocular allergies since it has been reported that approximately 50% of these patients have negative results on these tests [18-20]. A skin prick test examines the existence of sensitization to given allergens whereas RAST evaluates the amount of allergen specific IgE antibodies present in serum [21]. Tear cytology or conjunctival scrapping is useful in assessing the type and number of cells involved in conjunctival inflammation [6, 19].

The treatment options can range from purely non-pharmacological to concurrent use of pharmacological agents for supportive, prophylactic and pharmaceutical therapy. Although removal or avoidance of the offending allergens that incite allergy is the only absolute cure for allergic eye disease, when it is impossible, the clinician should recommend appropriate pharmacological treatment modalities. Thus, if non-pharmacologic management fails to mitigate the allergic response, the next step is to prescribe specific pharmacological agents, based on a comprehensive case history, as well as adequate knowledge of the clinicopathological features and differentials of allergic ocular surface disease [22]. The clinician may use pharmaceutical agents that prevent mast cell degranulation, block the histamine receptors, inhibit the release of arachidonic acid, inhibit T–lymphocyte activation, induces immunologic tolerance to the allergens, block the action of cyclooxygenase and inhibit Lipoxygenase pathway or combinations [23].

In this book, the basic concepts of immunology will be reviewed with emphasis on the lymphocyte activation, as well as IgE-mediated and T-lymphocyte mediated hypersensitivity response. The cells and mediators that play a crucial role in the pathomechanisms of ocular allergy will be discussed. Moreover, the clinical features and pathomechanisms of the specific types of allergic disorders of the ocular surface will be discussed, since such knowledge is critical to achieving success in the treatment and management of ocular allergy. Finally, treatment and management strategies including preventative measures, as well as the complications and prognosis of the allergic disorders of the ocular surface will be presented in detail.

References

[1]   Irkeç, M. and B. Bozkurt, Epithelial cells in ocular allergy. *Curr Allergy Asthma Rep,* 2003. 3(4): p. 352-7.

[2]   Bielory, L., et al., Treating the ocular component of allergic rhinoconjunctivitis and related eye disorders. *MedGenMed,* 2007. 9(3): p. 35.

[3]   Abelson, M., L. Smith, and M. Chapin, Ocular allergic disease: mechanisms, disease sub-types, treatment. *Ocul Surf,* 2003. 1(3): p. 127-49.

[4]   Manzouri, B., et al., Pharmacotherapy of allergic eye disease. *Expert Opin Pharmacother,* 2006. 7(9): p. 1191-200.

[5]   Leonardi, A., L. Motterle, and M. Bortolotti, Allergy and the eye. *Clin Exp Immunol,* 2008. 153 Suppl 1: p. 17-21.

[6]   Leonardi, A., C. De Dominicis, and L. Motterle, Immunopathogenesis of ocular allergy: a schematic approach to different clinical entities. *Curr Opin Allergy Clin Immunol,* 2007. 7(5): p. 429-35.

[7]   Reiss, J., et al., Allergic conjunctivitis. In: Pepose JS, Holland GN, Wilhelmus KR, editors. Ocular infection and immunity. 1996, St. Louis: *Mosby.* 345–58.

[8]   Pawankar, R., Inflammatory mechanisms in allergic rhinitis. *Curr Opin Allergy Clin Immunol,* 2007. 7(1): p. 1-4.

[9]   Chigbu, D.I., The pathophysiology of ocular allergy: a review. *Cont Lens Anterior Eye, 2009.* 32(1): p. 3-15; quiz 43-4.

[10] Leonardi, A., L. Motterle, and M. Bortolotti, Allergy and the eye. *Clin Exp Immunol,* 2008. 153 Suppl 1: p. 17-21.

[11] Berdy, G., Atopic keratoconjunctivitis (AKC). *Acta Ophthalmol Scand Suppl,* 1999(228): p. 7-9.

[12] Stahl, J.L., et al., Pathophysiology of ocular allergy: the roles of conjunctival mast cells and epithelial cells. *Curr Allergy Asthma Rep,* 2002. 2(4): p. 332-9.

[13] Leonardi, A., Pathophysiology of allergic conjunctivitis. *Acta Ophthalmol Scand Suppl,* 1999(228): p. 21-3.

[14] McGill, J., et al., Allergic eye disease mechanisms. *Br J Ophthalmol,* 1998. 82(10): p. 1203-14.

[15] Paulsen, F., Functional anatomy and immunological interactions of ocular surface and adnexa. *Dev Ophthalmol,* 2008. 41: p. 21-35.

[16] Pflugfelder, S. and M. Stern, Immunoregulation on the ocular surface: 2nd Cullen Symposium. *Ocul Surf,* 2009. 7(2): p. 67-77.

[17] Rosenwasser, L., et al., A comparison of olopatadine 0.2% ophthalmic solution versus fluticasone furoate nasal spray for the treatment of allergic conjunctivitis. *Allergy Asthma Proc.* 29(6): p. 644-53.

[18] Bonini, S., et al., Vernal keratoconjunctivitis. *Eye,* 2004. 18(4): p. 345-51.

[19] Bonini, S., Atopic keratoconjunctivitis. *Allergy,* 2004. 59 Suppl 78: p. 71-3.

[20] Bonini, S., A. Lambiase, and R. Sgrulletta, Allergic chronic inflammation of the ocular surface in vernal keratoconjunctivitis. *Curr Opin Allergy Clin Immunol,* 2003. 3(5): p. 381-7.

[21] Lambiase, A., et al., Prospective, multicenter demographic and epidemiological study on vernal keratoconjunctivitis: a glimpse of ocular surface in Italian population. *Ophthalmic Epidemiol.* 16(1): p. 38-41.

[22] Chigbu, D.I. and S. Sandrasekaramudaly-Brown, Ocular surface disease: a case of vernal keratoconjunctivitis. *Cont Lens Anterior Eye,* 2011. 34(1): p. 39-44.

[23] Chigbu, D.I., The management of allergic eye diseases in primary eye care. *Cont Lens Anterior Eye,* 2009. 32(6): p. 260-72.

Chapter 2

Structure, Function and Immunology of the Ocular Surface

The ocular surface and its adnexa are comprised of the cornea, conjunctiva, the main lacrimal gland, glands of the eyelids (meibomian and Molls), accessory lacrimal glands and the nasolacrimal system [1]. This chapter will focus on the ocular surface as it is composed of epithelium of the conjunctiva, limbus and cornea, and it is prone to allergic-induced tissue remodeling and damage.

The anatomy and physiology of the conjunctiva and cornea will be reviewed as well as the immunology of the ocular surface. A brief overview of the structure and physiology of the limbus is necessary, as it is most likely to be affected in chronic allergic diseases of the ocular surface. The epithelium of the ocular surface forms a physical barrier against the external environment and functions as a defensive front line of the innate immune system [2].

The conjunctiva is an immunologically active mucosal site; however, there are several regulatory mechanisms in place to control the immune response in order to prevent tissue damage [3]. Immunoregulation is a form of tolerance and modulatory mechanism that acts to control the innate and adaptive immune response to limit tissue damage after environmental insults [4]. The immunoregulatory mechanism of the ocular surface prevents acute inflammatory reactions on the ocular surface from progressing, as well as limiting activation of lymphocytes during periods of inflammation [3].

Structure and Function
of the Ocular Surface

The conjunctiva, an immunologically active tissue, is a semitransparent mucous membrane that lines the globe over the sclera and the inner surface of the eyelids. Histologically, the conjunctiva consists of the epithelium and the lamina propria. The structure of the epithelium varies from nonkeratinized, stratified, squamous epithelium to a stratified columnar epithelium (bulbar conjunctiva) [5, 6]. There are two to seven layers of epithelial cells that are joined together by desmosomes and tight junctions [6]. The conjunctiva stroma consists of collagen, fibroblasts, blood vessels, and immune cells [7]. The conjunctiva is a highly vascularized tissue with lymphatics that drains into the preauricular and submandibular lymph nodes [5, 8-10]. High endothelial venule (HEV) is a specialized post-capillary venule found in the conjunctiva. It expresses cell-surface adhesion molecules [7, 11]. The chemokines (CCL21) on the surface of HEV activates chemokine receptors, CCR7 on T-lymphocytes and chemokine receptor signaling leads to an increase in affinity of integrin (LFA-1) on T-lymphocyte for adhesion molecules (ICAM-1) on HEV [12]. HEV plays a role in regulating transmigration of lymphocytes into the ocular tissue [7, 11]. The conjunctival stem cells are distributed throughout the conjunctival but may be more concentrated in the fornices [13]. The conjunctival epithelium has numerous mucin-secreting goblet cells, and as such, it produces the mucous component of the tear film, which stabilizes the aqueous layer by providing a hydrophilic contact surface [6].

The limbus is an annulus of tissue, 1.5 mm wide, surrounding the cornea that acts as a junctional barrier separating the cornea and conjunctiva [14, 15]. It is the region where the conjunctival surface vessels terminate, leaving the cornea an avascular structure [5]. Histologically, the limbal conjunctiva consists of an epithelium and a stroma. The limbal conjunctival epithelium consists of 8 - 10 cell layers of epithelial cells. The epithelium of the limbal conjunctiva is continuous with the epithelium of the bulbar conjunctiva on one side and with the corneal epithelium on the other [15]. The adhesion complex of the cornea and limbal epithelial are similar [16]. The limbal conjunctiva lacks the goblet cells that are found in the bulbar and fornix conjunctival epithelium [15]. The basal cell of the limbal conjunctiva contains epithelial stem cells that are required for corneal wound repair whereas the stroma of the limbal conjunctiva contains numerous blood vessels supplied by or draining into the episcleral vessels. The constant shedding of the superficial ocular surface epithelial cells and their replacement by stem cells contributes to the ocular surface immune defense, as infected or damaged epithelial cells that could trigger an immune response are removed [5, 15]. The superficial marginal plexus that gives rise to the corneal arcades are found in the limbal conjunctival stroma. The corneal arcades supply blood to the peripheral cornea. The palisades of Vogt, a unique anatomical feature of the limbal conjunctiva adjacent to the cornea, consists of radially oriented channels in the stroma of the limbal conjunctiva with their associated blood vessels separated from one another by thickened ridges of epithelium [15]. It is of note that the stem cells reside in the limbal palisades of Vogt. The rich limbal vascular network of the palisades of Vogt provides nourishment to the metabolically active stem cells [14, 17]. Capillaries of the limbus have thicker endothelium and fewer fenestrations than those of the conjunctiva [18]. The limbal epithelium prevents the migration of conjunctival epithelial cells onto the cornea [19]. The limbus is richly invested with Langerhans' cells, which are capable of initiating an immune response following an encounter with antigen on the limbus. Thus, the limbus participates in immunosurveillance of the ocular surface [20, 21].

The cornea consists of five layers: epithelium, Bowman's layer, stroma, Descemet's membrane and endothelium. The epithelial layer is approximately 50 microns thick and is composed of stratified, non-keratinized cells arranged in five to seven cell layers with three distinctly different types of epithelial cells [22]. The three cells of the epithelial layer include superficial squamous, wing and basal cells [23]. Sensory nerve fibers derived from the ophthalmic division of the trigeminal nerve supply the cornea. The nerve fibers enter the peripheral cornea stroma and divide into smaller branches that penetrate the epithelium to form the intraepithelial sensory nerve plexus [24]. Corneal innervation is important for the maintenance of corneal structure and function [25]. The basal epithelial cell layer consists of columnar cells, and it secretes the basement membrane. It is attached to the basement membrane by a three dimensional structure termed the adhesion complex [26, 27]. The Bowman's layer is an anterior acellular zone that consists primarily of type I and III collagen fibrils and proteoglycans. The corneal stroma is about 500 microns thick and constitutes about 90% of the thickness of the entire cornea. It consists of a network of rigid, fibrillar collagen molecules and highly hydrated proteoglycan molecules [22]. The Descemet's membrane, a basement membrane, lies between the stroma and endothelium. It is composed of collagen type IV and laminin. The endothelium, a single cell layer, is the innermost layer of the cornea. It maintains corneal hydration and transparency [22, 28, 29].

The corneal epithelium, a stratified non-keratinized squamous epithelium with luminal junctions, provides a barrier to prevent external material such as dust, allergens and microorganism from entering the eye [30, 31]. Intercellular junctional complexes composed of tight junctions, adherens junctions, and desmosomes maintain the integrity of the corneal epithelial layer. The gap junctions provide for intercellular communication [32]. Adherens junctions (AJs) and tight junctions (TJs) play a vital role in the formation and maintenance of epithelial barriers [30]. TJ complex consists of transmembrane proteins (claudin; occludin), cytoplasmic or membrane-associated proteins (zonula occludens (ZO)-1, ZO-2, and ZO-3), and junctional adhesion molecules (JAM) [30, 32, 33]. Tight junctions link the cytoskeletons of adjacent epithelial cells, and as such, they contribute to the physiological barrier function of the corneal epithelium, as well as increase adhesion and stability [30, 34]. AJs complex consist of cadherins and catenins (α-catenin, β-catenin, p120 catenin) and it is positioned below the tight junctions [30]. Both AJs and TJs are firmly connected to the actin cytoskeleton. Because the barrier function of the corneal epithelium is susceptible to disruption by inflammation, chronic ocular allergic inflammation may disrupt the epithelial intercellular junctional complexes, which in turn, results in an alteration of the structure and function of the corneal epithelium [30]. The loss of conjunctival surface integrity due to the allergic inflammation-induced alteration in expression of AJs and TJs, could in turn lead to increased penetration of allergen and an exacerbation of the allergic response [34].

Immunology of the Ocular Surface

The ocular surface is exposed to the external environment, and as such, it is constantly under attack from non-pathogenic and pathogenic antigens. The ocular surface mucosal immunity utilizes innate and adaptive effector mechanisms present in tears and ocular surface to protect the ocular surface from damage [31]. Ocular surface epithelial cells are involved in initiating, mediating and regulating the innate and adaptive immune response of the ocular surface [35, 36].

Eye-associated lymphoid tissue (EALT) is an ocular surface immune protection system that consists of lymphoid tissue of the lacrimal gland, conjunctival-associated lymphoid tissue (CALT) and lacrimal drainage-associated lymphoid tissue (LDALT) [7]. CALT is the physiological protective tissue of the conjunctiva. CALT and conjunctival epithelium that consists of toll-like receptors (TLR) and tight junction between epithelial cells provide immune protection to the conjunctiva. EALT consists of diffuse lymphoid effector tissue and follicular lymphoid tissue [31]. Diffuse lymphoid effector tissue is the efferent arm of EALT. It consists of innate immune cells (dendritic cells, macrophages, neutrophils, mast cells), IgA$^+$plasma cells, and intraepithelial and lamina propria effector T-lymphocytes (CD4$^+$T- and CD8$^+$T-lymphocytes). Follicular organized lymphoid tissue, an afferent arm of EALT, is interspersed within the diffuse effector lymphoid tissue, and as such, both of them have the same topographical distribution. It consists of B cells, parafolicular T-cells associated with lymph vessels and HEV, and apical follicle-associated epithelium [7, 31, 37]. The main function of EALT is to maintain a balance between generation of immune tolerance and generation of immune-mediated ocular surface inflammatory process [7]. EALT favors immune tolerance by providing afferent (detecting antigen and generating immune reaction) and efferent (secretory IgA, regulatory T-lymphocytes, and immunosuppressive cytokines) immunological protection for the ocular surface [37].

EALT in the tarso-orbital zone of the palpebral conjunctiva supports immunosurveillance of the cornea, as it may act as an immunological windscreen wiper during blink action of the eyelid and as an immunological cushion during eye closure in sleep, which covers the cornea. Thus, EALT assists with immunosurveillance by providing the cornea with innate chemicals, upregulating pro-inflammatory factors from neutrophils to suppress microbial growth during sleep, and detect antigen and generate immunocompetent effectors [7, 31, 37].

Ocular surface epithelial cells play an important role in immune defense and inflammation, as well as in immunoregulation of the ocular surface. The innate immune cells (macrophages, dendritic cells, eosinophils, neutrophils, mast cells) and adaptive immune cells (B- and T-lymphocytes) are involved in host defense and inflammation [38]. T-lymphocytes mediate the cellular defense mechanism of the adaptive immune system whereas secretory IgA mediates the humoral defense mechanism of the adaptive immune system of the ocular surface [31].

Immune privilege at the ocular surface encompasses anatomical, physiological, and immunoregulatory mechanisms of the ocular surface. It prevents or resolves immune-mediated destruction of the ocular surface and maintains homeostasis [4, 39]. Immunoregulation of the ocular surface is controlled by afferent and efferent mechanisms. Regulating dendritic cell maturation; controlling production of pro-inflammatory cytokines by epithelium and dendritic cells via TLR; low level expression of adhesion molecules by vascular endothelial cells; mucin (forms a barrier against migration of inflammatory cells into the epithelium) production by epithelial and goblet cells; and release of neuropeptides by corneal sensory nerve fibers are afferent immunoregulatory mechanisms [3]. **Regulatory T-lymphocytes** (Tregs) and immunoregulatory cytokines such as transforming growth factor (TGF)-β and interleukin (IL)-10 control the efferent arm of immunoregulatory system of the ocular surface. Tregs suppress ocular surface inflammation by dampening T-lymphocyte priming in the lymph node and inhibiting Th1-, Th2-, and Th17-lymphocyte-mediated ocular surface inflammation [3, 4]. Additionally, immunoregulatory cytokines direct ocular surface antigen-presenting cells (APC) to promote activation and differentiation of regulatory T-lymphocytes in the regional lymph node [3]. TGF-β inhibits proliferation of injured or damaged corneal epithelial cells [40] via increasing the synthesis of tissue inhibitors of metalloproteinase (TIMP), which reduces the production of matrix metalloproteinase (MMP) [22, 29]. Furthermore, Th2-lymphocytes regulate immune tolerance via IL-4 and IL-5 that favor differentiation of B-lymphocytes into anti-inflammatory IgA$^+$plasma cells [37].

The tear film provides a physicochemical protection for the ocular surface. The physicochemical barrier of the epithelial-derived mucin layer that prevents adhesion and entrance of antigens supplements the flushing and diluting effects of the tear fluid and lid wiping combined with the action of protective proteins. Secreted antimicrobial peptides such as β-defensin 1- to -4, liver expressed antimicrobial peptide (LEAR)-1 and - 2, and cathelicidin (LL-37), lyzozyme, lactoferrin, secretory phospholipase A2 provide innate immune protection at the ocular surface [31]. Human β-defensin and LL-37 are expressed by ocular surface epithelial cells. These antimicrobial peptides are chemotactic for T-lymphocytes, neutrophils, monocytes, and mast cells [41, 42].

Complement regulatory protein such as decay accelerating factor (DAF; CD55) that disassembles C3/C5 convertase and protectin (CD59) that blocks assembly of membrane attack complex are expressed by ocular surface epithelial cells [43, 44]. Complement regulatory proteins prevent activation of complement, and as such, corneal epithelial cells are not susceptible to complement-mediated cytolysis and pro-inflammatory effects of complement components, C3a and C5a [39].

The cornea is an immunologically privileged tissue due to the lack of corneal vasculature and lymphatics, absence of mature antigen presenting cells in the central cornea, presence of vascular endothelium growth factor receptor in the corneal epithelium, and lack of Toll-like receptors (TLRs) on the apical layer of the corneal epithelium [45]. TLR1-10 is expressed on the ocular surface epithelium and stromal fibroblasts of the cornea. The immunosilent environment of the corneal epithelium could be attributed to the sub-apical corneal epithelia layer location of TLR4 and TLR5, which are expressed at the basal and wing cell layers. Thus, TLR-mediated innate immune response is triggered only when the epithelial barrier has been breached [46]. Vasoactive intestinal peptide (VIP) secreted by corneal sensory nerve fiber endings increases the production of immunoregulatory cytokines, while inhibiting the expression of pro-inflammatory cytokines and chemokines [3, 4]. The corneal epithelium expresses soluble vascular endothelium growth factor receptor-1 (VEGFR-1) and membrane-expressed VEGFR-3. VEGFR-1 and VEGFR-3 removes the angiogenic factors VEGF-A and VEGF-C respectively to reduce angiogenesis [4] and microvascular permeability, thereby limiting inflammatory cell infiltration into the ocular surface.

Fas ligand (FasL; CD95L) and tumor necrosis factor-related apoptosis-inducing ligand (TRAIL) are immunoregulatory processes that limit ocular surface damage by effector immune cells [3]. FasL and TRAIL are expressed on corneal cells including the epithelial cells. FasL (CD95L) prevents immune-mediated inflammation by inducing apoptosis of infiltrating neutrophil and activated lymphocytes that express the receptor for FasL (Fas; CD95). When TRAIL bearing corneal cells interacts with their respective receptors on inflammatory cells, it results in the apoptosis of the infiltrating cells [39]. Another immunoregulatory mechanism of the ocular surface involves interaction of programmed death ligand-1 (PD-L1) with PD-L1 receptors (PD-1) expressed on lymphocytes, natural killer cells, and macrophages [3, 47]. PD-L1 is upregulated on the ocular surface by pro-inflammatory cytokines. When PD-L1 interacts with PD-1, it leads to inhibition of T-lymphocyte proliferation and cytokine secretion [3, 39].

Ocular surface destruction or change in cytokine milieu involving increase in inflammatory cytokines can deregulate the physiological protective mucosal immune system of the ocular surface, since the above can skew antigen presentation in the direction of inflammatory response, as seen in ocular allergy. The deregulated resident lymphocytes of EALT play a role in immune-mediated inflammation of the ocular surface. **Pro-inflammatory cytokines are produced that are capable of activating ocular surface** epithelial cells to secrete pro-inflammatory factors (ICAM-1, cytokines, chemokines, and proteases), as well as upregulating costimulatory and MHC class II molecules on epithelial cells to present antigen to resident conjunctival T-lymphocytes. This results in the loss of natural ocular surface immune tolerance. Furthermore, stromal macrophages and fibroblasts secrete MMP that degrade stromal collagen and epithelial basement membrane [37]. Increased levels of MMP breaches the ocular surface epithelium; such breach allows antigens into the ocular surface subepithelial tissues to trigger activation of immature dendritic cells and conjunctival vascular endothelium [4]. Furthermore, pro-inflammatory cytokines can activate immature APCs on the cornea to express MHC class II molecules, CCR7 and CD80/CD86. There is also upregulation of adhesion molecules by epithelial cells, stromal fibroblasts, and vascular endothelium cells that result in recruitment of leukocytes into the ocular tissue [3]. Thus, activation of resident conjunctival lymphocytes, conjunctival vascular endothelium, ocular surface epithelial cells, and fibroblasts, as well as the influx of leukocytes, deregulates CALT leading to immune-mediated ocular surface inflammatory [7, 31].

The ocular surface epithelial cells located at the portals of allergen entry into the eye, produce inflammatory mediators (IL-1 α, TNF-α, and IL-6, and IL-8) and adhesion molecules (ICAM-1) that initiate allergic inflammation as well as trigger the recruitment of the inflammatory cells into the site of allergic inflammation. Thus, the immune mechanism of the ocular surface epithelium plays a role in ocular allergy [6].

References

[1] Paulsen, F., Functional anatomy and immunological interactions of ocular surface and adnexa. *Dev Ophthalmol,* 2008. 41: p. 21-35.

[2] Ueta, M. and S. Kinoshita, Innate immunity of the ocular surface. *Brain Res Bull,* 2010. 81(2-3): p. 219-28.

[3] Pflugfelder, S. and M. Stern, Immunoregulation on the ocular surface: 2nd Cullen Symposium. *Ocul Surf,* 2009. 7(2): p. 67-77.

[4] Stern, M.E., et al., Autoimmunity at the ocular surface: pathogenesis and regulation. *Mucosal Immunol,* 2010. 3(5): p. 425-42.

[5] Forrester, J.V., et al., Dendritic cell physiology and function in the eye. *Immunol Rev,* 2010. 234(1): p. 282-304.

[6]   Irkeç, M. and B. Bozkurt, Epithelial cells in ocular allergy. *Curr Allergy Asthma Rep,* 2003. 3(4): p. 352-7.

[7]   Knop, E. and N. Knop, The role of eye-associated lymphoid tissue in corneal immune protection. *J Anat,* 2005. 206(3): p. 271-85.

[8]   Donshik, P.C., W.H. Ehlers, and M. Ballow, Giant papillary conjunctivitis. *Immunol Allergy Clin North Am,* 2008. 28(1): p. 83-103, vi.

[9]   Elhers, W. and P. Donshik, Giant papillary conjunctivitis. *Curr Opin Allergy Clin Immunol,* 2008. 8(5): p. 445-9.

[10]   Donshik, P.C., Giant papillary conjunctivitis. *Trans Am Ophthalmol Soc,* 1994. 92: p. 687-744.

[11]   Knop, N. and E. Knop, Conjunctiva-associated lymphoid tissue in the human eye. *Invest Ophthalmol Vis Sci,* 2000. 41(6): p. 1270-9.

[12]   Murphy, K.P., Travers, P., Walport, M., T Cell-Mediated Immunity, in *Janeway's Immunobiology.* 2012, Garland Science: New York. p. 335-386.

[13]   Nagasaki, T. and J. Zhao, Uniform distribution of epithelial stem cells in the bulbar conjunctiva. *Invest Ophthalmol Vis Sci,* 2005. 46(1): p. 126-32.

[14]   Sanghvi, A. and S. Basti, Conjunctival transplantation for corneal surface reconstruction--case reports and review of literature. *Indian J Ophthalmol,* 1996. 44(1): p. 33-8.

[15]   Oyster, C.W., The Limbus and the Anterior Chamber, in The Human Eye: Structure and Function. 1999, Sinauer Associates, Inc: Sunderland, Massachusetts. p. 379-410.

[16]   Gipson, I.K., The epithelial basement membrane zone of the limbus. *Eye* (Lond), 1989. 3 (Pt 2): p. 132-40.

[17]   Ang, L.P. and D.T. Tan, Ocular surface stem cells and disease: current concepts and clinical applications. *Ann Acad Med Singa*pore, 2004. 33(5): p. 576-80.

[18]   Meyer, P.A., The circulation of the human limbus. *Eye* (Lond), 1989. 3 (Pt 2): p. 121-7.

[19]   Dua, H.S., The conjunctiva in corneal epithelial wound healing. *Br J Ophthalmol,* 1998. 82(12): p. 1407-11.

[20]   Cousins, S.W. and B.T. Rouse, Chemical Mediators of Ocular Inflammation In: Pepose JS, Holland GN, Wilhelmus KR, editors. *Ocular Infection and Immunity.* 1996, St Louis: Mosby. 50-70.

[21] Chandler, J.W., Ocular Surface Immunology In: Pepose JS, Holland GN, Wilhelmus KR, editors. *Ocular Infection and Immunity.* 1996., St Louis: Mosby. 104-111.

[22] Lim, M., et al., Growth factor, cytokine and protease interactions during corneal wound healing. *Ocul Surf,* 2003. 1(2): p. 53-65.

[23] Verma, A. Corneal Abrasion. Emedicine Ophthalmology 2009 February 25, 2010]; Available from: http://emedicine.medscape.com/article /1195402-overview.

[24] Pepose, J.S., Ubels, J.L., The Cornea, in Adler's Physiology of the Eye, W.M. Hart, Editor. 1992, *Mosby:* St. Louis. p. 29-70.

[25] Benitez-Del-Castillo, J.M., et al., Treatment of recurrent corneal erosion with substance P-derived peptide and insulin-like growth factor I. *Arch Ophthalmol,* 2005. 123(10): p. 1445-7.

[26] Chen, Y.T., et al., The cleavage plane of corneal epithelial adhesion complex in traumatic recurrent corneal erosion. *Mol Vis,* 2006. 12: p. 196-204.

[27] Dursun, D., et al., Treatment of recalcitrant recurrent corneal erosions with inhibitors of matrix metalloproteinase-9, doxycycline and corticosteroids. *Am J Ophthalmol,* 2001. 132(1): p. 8-13.

[28] Imanishi, J., et al., Growth factors: importance in wound healing and maintenance of transparency of the cornea. *Prog Retin Eye Res,* 2000. 19(1): p. 113-29.

[29] Klenkler, B., H. Sheardown, and L. Jones, Growth factors in the tear film: role in tissue maintenance, wound healing, and ocular pathology. *Ocul Surf,* 2007. 5(3): p. 228-39.

[30] Kimura, K., S. Teranishi, and T. Nishida, Interleukin-1beta-induced disruption of barrier function in cultured human corneal epithelial cells. *Invest Ophthalmol Vis Sci,* 2009. 50(2): p. 597-603.

[31] Knop, E. and N. Knop, Anatomy and immunology of the ocular surface. *Chem Immunol Allergy,* 2007. 92: p. 36-49.

[32] Schneeberger, E.E. and R.D. Lynch, The tight junction: a multifunctional complex. *Am J Physiol Cell Physiol,* 2004. 286(6): p. C1213-28.

[33] Yi, X., Y. Wang, and F.S. Yu, Corneal epithelial tight junctions and their response to lipopolysaccharide challenge. *Invest Ophthalmol Vis Sci,* 2000. 41(13): p. 4093-100.

[34] Ohbayashi, M., et al., The Role of Histamine in Ocular Allergy. *Adv Exp Med Biol,* 2010. 709: p. 43-52.

[35] Ma, P., et al., Human corneal epithelium-derived thymic stromal lymphopoietin links the innate and adaptive immune responses via TLRs and Th2 cytokines. *Invest Ophthalmol Vis Sci,* 2009. 50(6): p. 2702-9.

[36] Zheng, X., et al., Induction of Th17 differentiation by corneal epithelial-derived cytokines. *J Cell Physiol,* 2010. 222(1): p. 95-102.

[37] Knop, E. and N. Knop, Influence of the eye-associated lymphoid tissue (EALT) on inflammatory ocular surface disease. *Ocul Surf,* 2005. 3(4 Suppl): p. S180-6.

[38] Li, D., et al., Recent Advances in Mucosal Immunology and Ocular Surface Diseases, in Advances in Ophthalmology, S. Rumelt, Editor 2012. p. 49-78.

[39] Niederkorn, J.Y., Cornea: Window to Ocular Immunology. *Curr Immunol Rev,* 2011. 7(3): p. 328-335.

[40] Kuo, I.C., Corneal wound healing. *Curr Opin Ophthalmol,* 2004. 15(4): p. 311-5.

[41] McDermott, A.M., Defensins and other antimicrobial peptides at the ocular surface. *Ocul Surf,* 2004. 2(4): p. 229-47.

[42] Redfern, R.L., R.Y. Reins, and A.M. McDermott, Toll-like receptor activation modulates antimicrobial peptide expression by ocular surface cells. *Exp Eye Res,* 2011. 92(3): p. 209-20.

[43] Cocuzzi, E., et al., Release of complement regulatory proteins from ocular surface cells in infections. *Curr Eye Res,* 2000. 21(5): p. 856-66.

[44] Murphy, K.P., Travers, P., Walport, M., Innate Immunity: The First Lines of Defense, in Janeway's Immunobiology. 2012, Garland Science: New York. p. 37-74.

[45] Gilger, B.C., Immunology of the ocular surface. *Vet Clin North Am Small Anim Pract,* 2008. 38(2): p. 223-31, v.

[46] Lambiase, A., et al., Toll-like receptors in ocular surface diseases: overview and new findings. *Clin Sci* (Lond), 2011. 120(10): p. 441-50.

[47] Sharpe, A.H., et al., The function of programmed cell death 1 and its ligands in regulating autoimmunity and infection. *Nat Immunol,* 2007. 8(3): p. 239-45.

Chapter 3

Cells and Mediators in Allergic Ocular Surface Diseases

Adhesion Molecules

Adhesion molecules play a pivotal role in the recruitment of leukocytes to the site of inflammation. They mediate the interactions between leukocytes and endothelial cells during inflammatory responses by recruiting circulating leukocytes into the site of inflammation [1]. Additionally, chemokines stimulate epithelial cells to upregulate adhesion molecules and promote leukocyte adhesion, migration, accumulation, and activation [2].

The cell adhesion molecules are classified into three major families: (a) the integrins, (b) the selectins, and (c) the immunoglobulin gene superfamily [1, 3]. Very late activation antigen-4 (VLA-4) and lymphocyte function associated antigen-1 (LFA-1) are members of the integrin family. Intercellular adhesion molecule -1 (ICAM-1), ICAM-3 and vascular cell adhesion molecule-1 (VCAM-1) are members of the immunoglobulin gene superfamily [4].

LFA-1 plays a vital role in the extravasation of leukocytes. They bind to ICAM-1 and ICAM-2 to form strong adhesion between leukocytes and endothelial cells on inflamed endothelium [1].

The selectin family includes three adhesion molecules designated by the prefixes E (endothelial), P (platelet), and L (leukocyte) [5]. E-selectin (CD62E), expressed on the endothelium, mediates rolling of neutrophils on the endothelium. P-selectin (CD62P) is expressed on platelets and the endothelium. L-selectin (CD62L), found only on leukocytes, guides the exit of leukocytes by mediating the rolling of leukocyte along the endothelium [3, 5]. Activation of endothelium by LTB4, histamine or tumor necrosis factor (TNF)-α induces expression of P-selectin and E-selectin that act to initiate endothelium-leukocyte interaction, that results in the reversible binding of leukocytes to the vessel wall [1].

Five members of the immunoglobulin gene superfamily expressed by endothelial cells includes ICAM-1 (CD54), ICAM-2 (CD102), VCAM-1 (CD106), platelet-endothelial cell adhesion molecule-1 (PECAM-1; CD3l), and the mucosal vascular addressin cell adhesion molecule 1 (MAdCAM-1) [5]. ICAMs on the endothelium facilitate the tight adhesion of leukocytes to the endothelium [1, 3]. TNF-α induces the expression of adhesion molecules such as ICAM-1 and ICAM-2 [1]. Additionally, it has been shown that interferon gamma (IFN-γ) and interleukin (IL)-1β can induce the expression of ICAM-1[4]. ICAM-I, a ligand of LFA-1, expressed on mononuclear cells and granulocytes [2], plays an important role in homing and migration of neutrophils and eosinophils that are involved in the inflammatory process [6]. Additionally, lymphocytes, antigen presenting cells (APCs), fibroblasts, and epithelial cells can express ICAM-1. There is no expression of ICAM-1 in normal conjunctival epithelial cells. ICAM-1 is rapidly expressed on epithelial cells following the allergic reaction, and it facilitates the migration of inflammatory cells into the site of allergic inflammation [2]. ICAM-2 is expressed on endothelium and is involved in leukocyte adherence [5]. PECAM-1, found on endothelial cells, platelets and leukocytes, plays a role in the adhesion and transmigration of leukocytes [3, 5].

Vascular adhesion protein-1 (VAP-I), an endothelial adhesion molecule, plays a role in the adhesion and transmigration of lymphocytes [5, 7].

The expression of ICAM-1, E-selectin, and VCAM-1 has been demonstrated to be increased in ocular allergic diseases [2]. The process of allergen-induced accumulation of inflammatory mediators and cells into the site of allergic inflammation is a three-step process mediated by adhesion molecules [8].

Allergens

Allergens are small antigens that diffuse across the mucosal surface to induce predominantly Th2-lymphocyte mediated response [9]. House dust mites, mold, and pollen allergens have protease activity. Allergen source-derived proteases act as allergens and promoters of allergenicity [10]. House dust mite produces protease allergens with cysteine and serine protease activity [11]. Dermatophagoides pteronyssinus 1 (Der p 1) and Der p 3 have cysteine protease activity, whereas Der p 6 and Der p 9 allergens have serine protease activity [10]. The proteolytic enzymes released by allergens can disrupt the epithelial intercellular tight junctions, and as such, allow the access of the allergen into the conjunctival subepithelial layer where it is taken up by antigen-presenting cell (APC), such as dendritic cells [9, 11, 12]. Fecal pellets from house dust mite (Der p 1) destroy the barrier function of the epithelium. This allows allergens access to APC in the conjunctival subepithelial layer. The activated APC initiates production of Der p 1-specific Th2-lymphocyte and Der p 1-specific immunoglobulin E (IgE) [9, 13]. House dust mite-derived protease and serine activities could induce the release of proinflammatory cytokines (interleukin-6) and chemokines (interleukin-8), which in turn, attracts and/or activates inflammatory cells into the site of allergic response [11]. Furthermore, allergen can initiate ocular surface inflammation via oxidative stress [14]. Thus, allergenic-derived proteases play a role in the pathogenesis of allergic eye diseases, since it enhances the access of allergens to dendritic cells that promote the differentiation of naive T-lymphocytes into allergen-specific Th-lymphocytes [10].

Antibodies

Antibodies are immunoglobulins produced by B-lymphocytes in response to antigenic stimulation. They have the ability to react with specific antigens that stimulated their production [15, 16]. The antigen receptor of B-lymphocytes is also known as membrane immunoglobulin (mIg) or surface immunoglobulin (slg) [17]. The five classes of antibodies are immunoglobulin G (IgG), IgM, IgA, IgD, and IgE. Immunoglobulins are the effector molecules of the humoral immune system that participate in antibody-mediated immune reactions, such as preventing pathogen adherence (neutralization), promoting phagocytosis (opsonization), and activating the complement system. Thus, they protect the mucosal surfaces, tissues, and blood from infections by neutralizing the pathogen or promoting its elimination before it can establish a significant infection [18]. IgG is the main antibody in serum and non-mucosal surfaces, whereas IgA is the principal antibody in mucosal immunity. IgG is very efficient at opsonizing pathogens for engulfment by phagocytes and a strong activator of the complement system. IgA is an efficient neutralizing antibody on the epithelial surfaces. IgA is a less potent opsonin and a weak activator of complement [18]. Secretory IgA, a non-complement fixing immunoglobulin, is produced by lacrimal gland and conjunctiva. It plays a vital immunoregulatory role in the ocular surface and tears via prevention of infection and immune-mediated ocular surface inflammation [19, 20]. IgE is the major antibody that participates in immediate hypersensitivity reactions. It binds to two types of IgE specific Fc receptors. FcεRI found on mast cells, basophils and activated eosinophils bind IgE with high affinity. FcεRII present on B-lymphocytes, activated T-lymphocytes, monocytes, eosinophils, and follicular dendritic cells bind IgE with low affinity [9, 21]. IgA binds to FcαRI on eosinophils, neutrophils and macrophages. IgG binds to FcγRI, FcγRII, and FcγRIII receptors on macrophages, neutrophils, and eosinophils. B-lymphocytes, Langerhans cells, and mast cells also express FcγRII. FcγRIII is also expressed on natural killer cells and mast cells [18].

Antigen

Antigen is a substance or molecule, foreign to the host that can induce an immune response [22]. Antigen presentation to naive T-lymphocytes takes place in lymphoid tissues and is usually carried out by mature dendritic cells that have migrated from peripheral tissues due to exposure to a maturation stimulus [23]. Thymus-independent antigens do not require the help of T-lymphocytes to induce B-lymphocyte response, whereas thymus-dependent antigens need collaboration with T-helper lymphocytes to induce B-lymphocyte activation. Many antigens are thymus-dependent in nature [18, 23]. Although it is of note that normal conjunctival cells do not express antigens, inflamed conjunctival epithelial cells will express antigens [24].

Antigen Presenting Cells

Antigen presenting cells (APC) are cells (macrophages, B cells and dendritic cells) that are capable of taking up antigen, processing it and then presenting it to lymphocytes in a form they can recognize [25-27]. APCs bear costimulatory molecules or ligands that interact with costimulatory receptors on naïve T-lymphocytes to provide co-stimulatory signals during T-lymphocyte activation [28]. They link the innate and adaptive immune systems by producing cytokines, which enhance innate immunity and contribute to lymphocyte activation and function. They display antigen peptide-MHC complexes on their surface that are necessary for initiating immune responses [16, 29]. APCs are classified based on their level of constitutive expression of major histocompatibility complex (MHC) class II antigen. Professional APCs such as dendritic cells, macrophages, B-lymphocytes, and Langerhans cells express high levels of MHC II antigen and costimulatory molecules. Nonprofessional APCs such as vascular endothelial cells, epithelial cells, and fibroblast do not express costimulatory and MHC class II molecules but express them when induced by pro-inflammatory mediators [14, 30].

B-Lymphocytes

B-lymphocytes, produced in the bone marrow, express immunoglobulin (IgM and IgD) on cell surface membranes, which act as antigen receptors [18, 31]. Th-lymphocytes interact with B cells and help them to proliferate and differentiate into effector B-lymphocytes and memory B-lymphocytes. Plasma cells are the effector form of B-lymphocytes that secrete antibodies [16, 17, 32]. Plasma cells can survive for only days or weeks whereas others are long lasting and account for the persistence of antibody responses [18]. Plasma cells (terminally differentiated B-lymphocytes) are not capable of interacting with helper T-lymphocytes or responding to antigen because they have very low levels of surface immunoglobulin and lack MHC class II molecules. Plasmablasts are cells that have begun to secrete antibody but still possess many of the characteristics of activated B-lymphocytes that allow their interaction with T-lymphocytes. Thus, they express B7 co-stimulatory molecules and MHC class II molecules [18]. B-lymphocytes that produce cytokines are subdivided into effector and regulatory B-lymphocytes [33]. Regulatory B-lymphocytes (Breg) promote immune tolerance by secreting immunosuppressive cytokines that support regulatory T-lymphocyte (Treg) differentiation [33, 34]. Breg and Treg downregulates allergic diseases [35]. Effector B-lymphocytes secrete cytokines that amplify humoral and cellular immunity. B-lymphocytes primed by Th1-lymphocytes and antigen secrete interleukin (IL)-12 and interferon (IFN)-γ, whereas B-lymphocytes primed by Th2-lymphocytes and antigen secrete IL-4 and IL-13 [33].

Chemokines

Chemokines are a large family of structurally homologous, low molecular weight cytokines that attract and activate leukocytes [2]. Different types of cells release chemokines. They recruit monocytes, neutrophils, lymphocytes and other effector cells to the site of inflammation [1]. Thus, chemokines plays an important role in inflammation, cell trafficking, angiogenesis and wound healing [36]. The two broad groups of the chemokine family that act on different sets of receptors include CC chemokines and CXC chemokines. CC chemokines bind to CC chemokine receptors (CCR) whereas the CXC chemokines bind to CXC receptors (CXCR) [1].

Monocyte chemotactic protein-1 (MCP-1/ CCL2) produced by monocytes, macrophages, fibroblasts and keratinocytes acts on CCR2 receptors and plays a role in attracting monocytes, T-lymphocytes, and dendritic cells to the site of inflammation. It also activates macrophages and mast cells [1, 9].

Interleukin (IL)-8/CXCL8 is produced by monocytes, macrophages, fibroblasts, epithelial cells, and endothelial cells. It attracts neutrophils and naive T-lymphocytes to the site of inflammation. The receptors for CXCL8 are CXCR1 and CXCR2 [1].

CXCL10 produced by keratinocytes, monocytes, T-lymphocytes, fibroblasts, and endothelium, acts on CXCR3. They attract resting T-lymphocytes and monocytes to the site of inflammation. They play a role in promoting Th1-mediated immunity [1].

T-lymphocytes, endothelial cells, and platelets produce CCL5 (RANTES) that acts on CCR1, 3, 5 [2]. Regulated on activation normal T-cell expressed and secreted (RANTES) attracts monocytes, T-lymphocytes, basophils, eosinophils, and dendritic cells. It plays a role in triggering the degranulation of basophils, activating T-lymphocytes, and inducing chronic inflammation [1].

CCL11 (Eotaxin), produced by endothelial cells, monocytes, epithelial cells, and T-lymphocytes, acts on CCR3. It attracts eosinophils, monocytes, and T-lymphocytes to the site of allergic inflammation [1]. Eotaxin is a potent chemotactic cytokine for eosinophils [2].

CXCL8 induces neutrophils to leave the bloodstream and migrate into the surrounding tissues whereas CCL2 induces the migration of monocytes from the bloodstream into the surrounding tissue where they become tissue macrophages [1]. Under allergen-induced ocular surface inflammation, inflammatory cells, stimulated epithelial cells, fibroblasts and vascular endothelial cells in the conjunctiva produce chemokines [37].

Complement

The complement system consists of a large number of different plasma proteins that interact with one another to opsonize pathogens, recruit inflammatory and immunocompetent cells, and destroy pathogens. The three pathways of the complement system include classical, lectin, and alternate pathways. During complement activation, C3 convertase cleave C3 to generate C3b and C3a. The binding of C3b to C3 convertase yields C5 convertase that produces C5a and C5b. C3b is the main effector molecule of the complement system whereas C5a is the most potent inflammatory peptide of the complement system. The complement fragments C3a and C5a are peptide mediators of inflammation that are capable of producing local inflammatory responses by acting directly on local blood vessels, stimulating an increase in blood flow, and increased binding of phagocytes to vascular endothelial cells. Additionally, they are capable of inducing smooth muscle contraction and increased vasopermeability [1, 38]. Moreover, C5a and C3a act on vascular endothelial cells to induce expression of adhesion molecules as well as activate mast cells to release pro-allergic and pro-inflammatory mediators [1, 39].

Co-Stimulatory Molecules and Receptors

Co-stimulatory molecules or ligands are cell surface proteins on APCs that interact with cell surface (co-stimulatory) receptors on naïve T-lymphocytes, to transmit a signal that is required along with antigen to induce T-lymphocyte activation [40, 41]. The co-stimulatory molecules B7 (B7.1 (CD80) and B7.2 (CD86)) are rapidly upregulated on memory B-cells, and as such, they enhance the brisk and robust nature of the secondary response [36].

CD28 is a co-stimulatory receptor on the surface of all naïve T-lymphocytes and binds to co-stimulatory ligand B7, which are expressed mainly on APCs such as dendritic cells [40, 42]. CD28 signaling aids antigen-dependent T-lymphocyte activation mainly by promoting T-lymphocyte proliferation, cytokine production, and cell survival [28]. CD28 amplifies or stabilizes the signal through the T cell receptor (TCR), a signal that is crucial for IL-2 production. It is of note that CD28 is also expressed on activated T-lymphocytes [23].

Cytotoxic T-Lymphocyte Antigen 4 (CTLA-4) is another CD28-related protein that has a high affinity for B7 molecules. The interaction between CTLA-4 (CD152) and B7 molecules will inhibit the proliferation of activated T-lymphocytes. CD28 interaction with co-stimulatory ligands on APC will enhance TCR signaling whereas CTLA-4 interaction with the same co-stimulatory ligand will cause an inhibition of the TCR signaling [40, 42]. CTLA-4 acts to keep T-lymphocytes under control and as such, it prevent responses of T-lymphocytes to self antigen [23].

OX40, a co-stimulatory receptor, expressed on activated T-lymphocytes and its ligand (OX40L) expressed on activated dendritic cells provide OX40-OX40L interactions that enhances T-lymphocyte survival and proliferation [43]. OX40L expression has been reported to be critical for the ability of TSLP-activated dendritic cells to trigger naïve T-lymphocytes to differentiate into Th2-lymphocytes that produce IL-4, IL-5, and IL-13, and in addition TNF-α [44]. OX40 and OX40L play a major role in the generation and maintenance of Th-lymphocyte memory [45]. Thus, they play a role in sustaining T-lymphocyte response [43].

Several studies have demonstrated that the CD28/CD86 costimulatory pathway is required for allergen-induced eosinophil recruitment, Th2-lymphocyte cytokine production and local production of IgE in allergic inflammation [40].

Cytokines

Cytokines are low molecular weight, highly potent secreted proteins that mediate cell division, inflammation, cytotoxicity, differentiation, migration, and repair. Interleukins (ILs), cytokines made by leukocytes, act as communicators between leukocytes. They are more than 30 interleukins. Other cytokine families include colony stimulating factors (support proliferation of hematopoietic precursors), tumor necrosis factor (cytotoxic towards transformed cell types), and interferons (interfere with viral replication) [36].

IL-1 (IL-1α and IL-1β), a cytokine produced by monocytes, macrophages, dendritic cells, and endothelial cells, plays an essential role in the initiation and coordination of host defenses in response to trauma, infection, and inflammation. IL-1 increases the expression of chemokine and adhesion molecules on endothelium; activates macrophages to release IL-1,-6,-8, TNF, GM-CSF and PGE2; increases lymphocyte proliferation, and plays a role in the immunopathogenesis of allergic disease [36, 46]. IL-1beta is capable of stimulating the release of VEGF from conjunctival fibroblast, and as such, it plays an important role in allergic eye disorders [47].

IL-2, produced by CD4$^+$T-lymphocytes and CD8$^+$T lymphocytes promotes the proliferation of activated T- and B-lymphocytes [36, 43, 48].

IL-4, produced by Th2-lymphocytes and mast cells, induces differentiation of T-lymphocytes into Th2-lymphocytes; stimulates proliferation of activated B-lymphocytes; upregulates MHC class II molecule expression on B-lymphocytes; downregulates IL-12 production; and induces the production of IgG1 and IgE [36, 43]. IL-13 is produced by Th2-lymphocytes and mast cells. It inhibits activation and cytokine secretion by macrophage; upregulates MHC class II and CD23 (FcεRII) on B-lymphocytes; induces the synthesis of IgG1 and IgE; and induces the expression of VCAM-1 on endothelium [36]. IL-4 is produced by mast cells in allergic conjunctivitis and predominantly produced by Th2-lymphocytes in chronic ocular allergy [49]. IL-4 and IL-13 can induce tissue remodeling by stimulating conjunctival fibroblast to proliferate and produce VEGF, which culminates in papillary formation with new vessels [47]. Additionally, IL-4 and IL-13 augments the buildup of collagen at the site of allergic inflammation by increasing the production of tissue inhibitors of metalloproteinase (TIMP)-1 and downregulating the expression of matrix metalloproteinase (MMP)-1 [50]. Thus, they may play an important role in the pathogenesis of ocular allergic disorders.

IL-5, produced by Th2-lymphocytes and mast cells, induces the activation and proliferation of eosinophils [51]. It also promotes the proliferation and differentiation of allergen-activated B-lymphocytes as well as augments the production of IgA. Th2-lymphocytes, monocyte, macrophage, and dendritic cells produce IL-6. IL-6 enhances the proliferation of B- and T-lymphocytes [36].

IL-9 is secreted by T-lymphocytes, eosinophils, mast cells and neutrophils [52]. IL-9 synergizes with IL-4 in producing IgG1 and IgE [36, 53]. It stimulates mast cells to secrete cytokine and protease, as well as stimulates epithelial cells to express chemokines to enhance eosinophil and T-lymphocyte infiltration [53]. Furthermore, IL-9 stimulates the expression of the high-affinity IgE receptor on mast cells [54]. The IL-9 gene is located on chromosome 5 (5q31-35), a region that contains genes encoding IL-3, IL-4, IL-5, IL-13, and granulocyte- macrophage colony-stimulating factor [52, 54]. Thus, IL-9 can augment remodeling and perpetuate chronic inflammation in allergic conditions [52].

IL-10, produced by monocytes and regulatory T-lymphocytes, is a cytokine synthesis inhibitory factor that suppresses T-lymphocyte mediated reactions through inhibition of MHC class II molecule and B7 co-stimulatory ligand expression on dendritic cells and macrophages [36]. Because it inhibits the release of cytokine it could attenuate allergic conjunctivitis [55]. IL-12, produced by monocytes, macrophage, and dendritic cells, stimulates the synthesis of IFN-γ and the differentiation of naive CD4$^+$T-lymphocytes into Th1-lymphocytes. IL-16, produced by T-lymphocytes and mast cells, is a chemoattractant for CD4$^+$T-lymphocytes, monocyte and eosinophils [36].

IL-17 is a cytokine produced by neutrophils, NK cells, Th17- and Tc17-lymphocytes [36, 43]. IL-17 is proinflammatory in nature and triggers the secretion of proinflammatory cytokines and chemokines from epithelial cells, endothelial cells, and fibroblasts [36, 56]. Because IL-17 is produced by both innate and adaptive cells, it creates a link between innate and adaptive immunity [57, 58]. IL-21, produced by activated CD4$^+$T-lymphocytes, plays a role in inducing the proliferation of natural killer (NK) cells, T- and B-lymphocytes via interactions with IL-21 receptors on NK cells, T- , and B-lymphocytes [59]. IL-21 receptors are also expressed on dendritic cells, macrophages, and epithelial cells [60]. IL-21 is involved in chronic inflammatory and allergic diseases [61]. IL-22 is a cytokine produced by Th22-lymphocytes with receptors expressed on non-immune cells, such as epithelial cells [62, 63]. Th17-lymphocytes and NK cells also produce IL-22 [43]. IL-22 induces proinflammatory responses via the production of cytokines and chemokines, and as such, it is involved in the pathogenesis of many inflammatory skin diseases [48, 60]. Because IL-22 receptors are expressed on epithelial cells, IL-22 could be involved in mucosal immunity [60].

IL-23, produced by dendritic cells, induces the release of proinflammatory cytokines such as IL-1, IL-6, and TNF-α by macrophages, as well as the clonal expansion and survival of Th17-lymphocytes [36]. IL-33, expressed mainly by fibroblasts, epithelial, and endothelial cells, is a potent activator of the innate immune system [36, 64]. As a potent activator of mast cells, it can induce degranulation and the subsequent production of pro-inflammatory cytokines. Additionally, it is capable of driving dendritic cells to mediate the differentiation of naïve CD4$^+$T-lymphocytes into Th2-lymphocytes, as well as the production of cytokines such as IL-4, IL-5 and IL-13 [64]. IL-35, produced by regulatory T-lymphocytes, is an immunosuppressive cytokine that suppresses the effects on Th1-, Th2-, and Th17-lymphocytes [36].

Granulocyte-macrophage colony stimulating-factor (GM-CSF) is produced by T-lymphocytes, macrophages, fibroblasts, mast cells, and endothelial cells. It stimulates the growth of progenitors of monocytes, neutrophils, eosinophils and basophils [36]. It activates macrophage and induces the differentiation of macrophages into dendritic cells [43].

Interferon (IFN)-β is produced by fibroblasts, whereas IFN-α is produced by leukocytes and dendritic cells. IFN-α and IFN-β are type 1 IFNs, produced in response to viral infection. IFN-α/β signaling is critical for enhancing the activation and proliferation of CD8+T-lymphocytes, as well as the generation of memory CD8+T-lymphocyte [36, 65]. IFN-γ, produced by Th1-lymphocytes, CD8+T-lymphocytes, and Natural Killer cells, activate macrophages as well as increase the expression of MHC class I and class II molecules on macrophages [43].

Transforming growth factor (TGF)-beta, an immunosuppressive or immunoregulatory cytokine, is involved in the regulation of immune response [66]. It is secreted by monocytes, macrophages, mast cell, and regulatory T-lymphocytes. It induces the synthesis of IgA [36]. TGF-β inhibits the proliferation and differentiation of Th1-, Th2-, and Th17-lymphocytes [56]. It is of note that not all TGF-β effects are immunosuppressive in nature, as it is capable of producing proinflammatory effects by activating neutrophils [43].

Tumor necrosis factor (TNF) is a multifunctional proinflammatory cytokine. TNF-α is produced by monocytes, macrophages, dendritic cells, mast cell, and T-lymphocytes, whereas TNF-β is secreted by Th1-lymphocytes and cytotoxic T-lymphocytes [36]. TNF-α is a major mediator of acute inflammatory responses. It triggers the recruitment of neutrophils and monocytes to the site of inflammatory reaction by inducing the expression of adhesion molecules on vascular endothelial cells, as well as enhancing chemokine synthesis by epithelial cells, endothelial cells, and macrophages [2]. TNF-β (lymphotoxin) activates macrophages and neutrophils, as well as destroys fibroblast and tumor cells [43].

Dendritic Cells

Dendritic cells (DCs) are APCs that detect and present antigen to T-lymphocyte, which in turn culminates in triggering an adaptive immune response [17, 67]. The processing and presentation of antigen by DCs downregulates chemokine receptor, CCR6 and upregulates the expression of costimulatory molecules (CD80 and CD86) and CCR7 that directs activated DCs to regional lymph nodes [14, 68].

DCs arise from both myeloid and lymphoid progenitors within the bone marrow [43].

Myeloid (conventional) DCs express Toll-like receptor (TLR)-1 through TLR-6 and TLR-8 [69]. Mature conventional dendritic cells express MHC proteins and co-stimulatory molecules for priming naive T-lymphocytes [43]. Thus, mature dendritic cells play a crucial role in linking the innate and adaptive immune systems, since they can present antigens to naive T-lymphocytes, which in turn results in T-lymphocyte activation [17]. Immature dendritic cells express most of the TLRs; however, they do not bear many of the cell-surface molecules [43].

Plasmocytoid DCs express intracellular receptors TLR-7 and TLR-9. Although they are sentinels for viral infections and secrete large amounts of type I interferons, they are less efficient in activating naive T-lymphocytes [43, 69, 70].

Eosinophils

Eosinophils, granulocytic leukocytes originating in bone marrow, contain arginine-rich basic proteins. They play a role in the development and progression of inflammatory reactions in ocular allergy. Eosinophils secrete enzymes, cytokines, chemokines, lipid mediators and toxic granule proteins (eosinophil-derived cytotoxic proteins). The enzymes secreted by eosinophils include eosinophil peroxidase, eosinophil collagenases, and matrix metalloproteinase-9. Eosinophil peroxidase triggers histamine release from mast cells whereas eosinophil collagenases play a role in remodeling connective tissue matrix. MMP-9 degrades extracellular matrix protein. Eosinophil major basic protein is a toxic protein released by eosinophils that trigger histamine release from mast cells, as well as cause damage to the cornea in chronic allergic conditions. Additionally, toxic proteins such as eosinophil cationic protein and eosinophil-derived neurotoxin are known to be neurotoxic. Eosinophils secrete chemokines with Th2-lymphocyte chemoattractive properties such as CCL2, CCL11, CCL17, and CXCL8 [9, 71]. The cytokines secreted by eosinophils include IL-4, IL-6, IL-12, IL-13, and IL-25 [71].

Although eosinophils do not express Fc receptors in their non-activated state, they can express Fc receptors following activation by cytokines and chemokines. Thus, eosinophils will degranulate to release its mediators when allergens induce cross-linking of IgE bound to FcεRI on the eosinophil surface

[9]. Additionally, activated eosinophils express MHC II molecules and co-stimulatory molecules CD86 and CD40, and as such, they are capable of presenting antigen to naive or activated CD4$^+$T-lymphocytes [71, 72].

Chemokines, adhesion molecules and cytokines are involved in the recruitment of eosinophils to the site of inflammation in allergic eye diseases [73, 74]. Although eosinophils are not present in the normal conjunctiva, they are over-expressed in the conjunctiva of patients with chronic ocular allergy [2].

Epithelial Cells

Epithelium represents a physical barrier that protects against the intrusion of antigens through the function of adherens junctions and tight junctions that play a vital role in the formation and maintenance of epithelial barriers [12, 75]. The epithelial cells participates in innate and adaptive immunity [2]. Epithelial cells, which are located at the portals of allergen entry into the eye, act as a mechanical barrier to prevent entry of antigens into the eye, as well as actively participate in regulating allergic inflammation of the ocular surface via expression of cytokines, chemokines and adhesion molecules. These mediators promote the influx of eosinophils and T-lymphocytes into the site of allergic inflammation [2, 76, 77]. Histamine can stimulate conjunctival epithelial cells to secrete RANTES, eotaxin, CCL2, CXCL8, IL-6, and TNF-α [2]. Conjunctival and limbal epithelial cells express CD40 [2, 78], and IFN-γ and TNF-α has been shown to upregulate the expression of CD40 in ocular surface epithelial cells [2]. Thus, epithelial cells play an important role in ocular surface inflammation seen in patients with allergic eye disease.

Fibroblast

Fibroblast, a cell that produces extracellular matrix (ECM), plays an important role in providing structural support, as well as acting as sentinel cells of the immune system by producing pro-inflammatory mediators in response to inflammation [79]. It is an immune modulator of ocular allergic disorders. IL-4 and IL-13 stimulates corneal fibroblasts to express chemokines (eotaxin and thymus- and activation-regulated chemokine (TARC or CCL17), matrix metalloproteinase, and adhesion molecules (VCAM-1 and ICAM-1).

TARC is a potent chemoattractant for Th2-lymphocytes. It is of note that IL-4 and IL-13 induces the production of ECM and proliferation of conjunctival fibroblasts, which in turn contributes to the formation of giant papillae in chronic ocular allergy [80, 81]. Conjunctival fibroblasts promote allergic inflammation in the ocular surface by producing chemokines, cytokines, and adhesion molecules that facilitate the persistence of inflammatory cells at the site of allergic inflammation [50]. Additionally, TGF-β, IL-1β, IL-4 and IL-13 stimulates conjunctival fibroblasts to produce vascular endothelial growth factor (VEGF), which in turn, plays a role in the formation of giant papillae containing newly formed vessels in chronic ocular allergy [47, 82]. Thus, corneal and conjunctival fibroblasts contribute to tissue remodeling in allergic eye diseases.

Growth Factors

Growth factors modulate cellular growth, proliferation, and differentiation. Growth factors such as epidermal growth factor (EGF), fibroblast growth factor (FBF), and nerve growth factor (NGF) modulate the proliferation and differentiation of epithelial cells [83]. EGF, FBF, platelet-derived growth factor (PDGF), and transforming growth factor beta 1 (TGFβ-1) are fibrogenic factors that induce growth of fibroblast, and as such, they play a role in the pathomechanisms of VKC [47, 84]. TGF-β1 is involved in fibroblast proliferation and collagen synthesis in allergic eye diseases. Thus, TGF-β plays a role in regulating allergic inflammation and tissue remodeling in ocular allergy [47, 85]. Vascular endothelial growth factor (VEGF), a potent multifunctional cytokine, is involved in microvascular permeability, and it contributes to the development of new vessels in ocular allergy. VEGF is produced by human mast cells [47]. VEGF is involved in the fibrovascular proliferation that plays a role in the development of giant papillae, and as such, it plays a role in tissue remodeling in ocular allergy [86]. NGF induces mast cell degranulation and mediator release; modulates the proliferation of epithelial cells; and suppresses leukotriene C4 formation from eosinophils [83]. Lambiase and colleagues reported that patients with VKC have increased circulating NGF and they were able to demonstrate a direct correlation between NGF levels and number of mast cells in the inflamed conjunctiva [87]. These growth factors participate in the pathogenesis of chronic ocular allergy such as VKC [84].

Histamine

Histamine, a major vasoactive mediator stored in mast cells and basophils, is synthesized by the decarboxylation of the amino acid L-histidine by the enzyme histidine decarboxylase [88]. Histamine exerts its biological effects by interacting with four G-protein coupled receptors, classified as H1R-H4R [84]. H1R, H2R and H4R play a major role in allergic eye diseases [12]. The effect of histamine on H1R (H1 receptors) in the conjunctiva results in vasodilation, increased vasopermeability, pruritus, recruitment of inflammatory cells, fibroblast proliferation, and cytokine secretion. Histamine effects on the H2R result in increased vasopermeability, mucous discharge, and proliferation of cytokine production [12, 89]. The H4R are expressed on mast cells, eosinophils, T-lymphocytes, and dendritic cells [12], and as such, when histamine binds to H4R it may initiate the recruit of mast cells, eosinophils, dendritic cells and T-lymphocytes into conjunctival tissue. Thus, H4R is involved in chemotaxis of immune cells, cytokine and chemokine release, and adhesion molecule expression [12, 90]. Additionally, H4R may play a role in maintaining barrier function of the conjunctival epithelial cells in an allergic response, and as such, it maintains the integrity of the conjunctival barrier in the presence of allergen. However, histamine signaling via H1R or H2R may promote disruption of the barrier function of the conjunctival epithelium [12]. Histamine released following mast cell degranulation affects conjunctival blood vessels, nerve endings, epithelial cells and fibroblasts [89]. Furthermore, histamine stimulates conjunctival fibroblasts and epithelial cells to produce and express pro-inflammatory cytokines, chemokines, and adhesion molecules, which plays a role in conjunctival remodeling in ocular allergy [85]. Thus, histamine is a potent mediator that accounts for the majority of signs and symptoms of the allergic reaction [91, 92].

Langerhans Cells

Langerhans' cells are professional APCs [93]. The mature Langerhans cells are MHC class II-positive with CD80$^+$ and CD86$^+$, whereas immature Langerhans cells are MHC class II-negative with CD80$^-$ and CD86$^-$ molecules. They are immature dendritic cells that do not initially express co-stimulatory activity, and as such, they are unable to interact with antigenic-specific T-lymphocytes. When Langerhans cells take up antigen, they migrate to the regional lymph nodes where they differentiate into dendritic cells that express co-stimulatory B7 molecules and adhesion molecules, which enable them to interact with antigen-specific T-lymphocytes [43]. The most important APCs on the ocular surface of dendritic origin are Langerhans cells [2]. Clinical studies have suggested that interaction of CD86 on Langerhans cells with T lymphocytes mediates the development of the Th2-type immune response [94]. Langerhans cells are concentrated in the epithelium of the conjunctiva, limbus and peripheral cornea [68]. They regulate ocular surface immunity and link innate and adaptive effector mechanism in ocular surface disorders such as ocular allergy [20].

Leukotrienes

Leukotriene (LT), a potent inflammatory mediator formed from the lipoxygenase pathway of arachidonic acid metabolism, plays a role in the pathogenesis of allergic eye disorders [95]. LTB4, LTC4, LTD4 and LTE4 are released by mast cells [95], whereas LTC4, LTD4 and LTE4 are released by eosinophils [9]. Leukotrienes can cause smooth muscle contraction, increased vasopermeability, and increased mucus secretion [9]. Studies have shown an increase in the production of LTC4 following FcγRI and FcεRI aggregation, although LTC4 generation was more with IgE cross linking [96]. The action of leukotrienes on the conjunctiva may contribute to the presence of the characteristic manifestations of ocular allergy, such as excessive mucous secretion, conjunctival hyperemia and chemosis [97-99].

Macrophage

Macrophage, a mature form of monocyte found in almost all tissues, is a long-lived cell that performs many diverse functions during the innate immune response [17].

Monocytes are the precursor of the tissue macrophages. GM-CSF and IL-4 stimulates the monocytes to differentiate into dendritic cells, whereas the macrophage colony-stimulating factor (M-CSF) induces monocytes to differentiate into macrophages [1]. Macrophages that have a few or no MHC class II molecules on their surface and do not express B7 are resting macrophages. These cells express both MHC class II molecules and B7 when their receptors are involved in ingesting microorganisms by phagocytosis. The receptors include mannose receptor, scavenger receptor, complement receptor, and TLR that act as phagocytic receptors, as well as signal for the secretion of proinflammatory cytokines that recruit and activate more phagocytes [1, 43].

Macrophages are involved in the innate and adaptive immune process. In the innate immune system, macrophages play a protective role in phagocytosis, which in turn, triggers the activated macrophage to release chemokines and cytokines that aid in combating infection. In the adaptive immune system, macrophages can act as APC by presenting antigen to induce the activation of naïve T-lymphocytes. Tissue macrophages secrete cytokines that induce vasodilation and changes in the endothelial cells of the blood vessel walls at the site of infection and inflammation. These changes lead to leukocyte-endothelium interaction that culminates in the movement of leukocytes, such as neutrophils and monocytes, into the site of infection and inflammation [1].

Major Histocompatibility Complex

Major Histocompatibility Complex (MHC) is a cell surface recognition structure that plays a role in transporting processed antigen in the form of a complex to T-lymphocytes. The two major classes include MHC class I molecule and MHC class II molecule [16, 100]. The expression of MHC class I and II molecules are upregulated during innate and adaptive immune responses [2]. The polygenic and polymorphic nature of MHC makes it difficult for pathogens to evade immune responses [101]. Almost all nucleated cells express MHC class I molecules. Non-nucleated cells express little or no MHC class I molecules, and as such, when infected they can escape destruction by cytotoxic T-lymphocytes. MHC class I molecules present antigen in the form of peptides to $CD8^+$T-lymphocytes. B-lymphocytes, dendritic cells, and macrophages express MHC class II molecules. MHC class II molecules present antigen to $CD4^+$T-lymphocytes. The expression of MHC class I and MHC class II molecules are controlled by cytokines [102]. In humans, MHC is located on chromosome 6 and it contains more than 200 human leukocyte antigen (HLA) genes. HLA-A, -B and -C are class I α-chain genes. HLA-DR, -DP and -DQ, expressed on dendritic cells, B-lymphocytes and macrophages, are class II-α and β-chain genes [2, 102].

Mast Cells

Mast cells originate from hematopoietic stem cells and differentiate under the influence of stem cell factor [103]. The major factors for mast cell growth and development include stem-cell factor (SCF), IL-3, IL-4 and IL-9 [9]. Mast cells are mostly located in high concentrations in vascularized connective tissues just beneath epithelial surfaces [18]. Mast cells are involved in allergy and autoimmunity [9, 104].

In the normal conjunctiva, the mast cells are concentrated in the conjunctival substantia propria [105-107]. Although the healthy human conjunctiva has been estimated to contain more than 10,000 mast cells/mm^3 located in the substantia propria, the number increases in the chronic forms of ocular allergy with mast cells located in the epithelium and substantia propria of the conjunctiva [12]. Mast cells play a pivotal role in initiating the inflammatory cascade in allergic eye disease [84]. Mast cells express FcεRI and FcγR on their cell surface, which enables them to bind IgE and IgG respectively [84, 104]. Mast cell FcγR include activating and inhibitory receptors [104].

Immunohistochemical studies have demonstrated the presence two types of mast cells. Tryptase-positive (MC$_T$) mast cells contain tryptase. Chymase-positive (MC$_{TC}$) mast cells contain both tryptase and chymase [98]. MC$_{TC}$ mast cells expresses IL-4, a cytokine that plays a key role in allergy promoting T-lymphocyte growth, inducing IgE production from B cells, upregulating adhesion molecules and regulating Th2-lymphocyte differentiation [40].

Mast cells are activated via crosslinking of the high affinity IgE receptor (FcεRI) or non-IgE-mediated activation through complement receptors or TLR activation, resulting in degranulation and release of histamine, leukotrienes, proteases, prostaglandins, chemokines and cytokines [108, 109]. The preformed mediators include histamine, serotonin, heparin, neutral proteases (tryptase and chymase, carboxypeptidase, cathepsin G), major basic protein, acid hydrolases, peroxidase, and phospholipases [108]. Mast cell degranulation also leads to the release of pro-fibrogenic and pro-fibrolytic mediators. Histamine has pro-fibrogenic potential, since it can stimulate fibroblast proliferation whereas mast cell proteases (pro-fibrolytic mediators) can degrade collagen types IV and V, laminin and fibronectin [50]. Tryptase and chymase can activate matrix-degrading metalloproteinases to break down tissue matrix proteins, causing tissue destruction [9]. Lipid mediators include LTB4, LTC4, prostaglandin (PG) E2, PGD2, platelet-activating factor (PAF). The cytokines released includes TNF-α, TGF-β, IFN-α, IFN-β, IFN-γ, IL-1α,

IL-1β, IL-3, IL-4, IL-5, IL-6, IL-8, IL-9, IL-10, IL-11, IL-12, IL-13, IL-15, IL-16, IL-18, IL-25, and SCF. Chemokines such as CXCL8, CCL2, CCL3, CCL5, CCL7, CCL11, CCL13, and CCL19 are released following activation of mast cells. The growth factors include bFGF, VEGF, and NGF [108]. It is of note that TNF-α activates endothelial cells, causing an increased expression of adhesion molecules, which promotes the influx of leukocyte into the site of allergic inflammation [9]. The mediators released upon mast cell activation play a major role in the acute and chronic forms of ocular allergy.

Matrix Metalloproteinases

Matrix metalloproteinases (MMP) are extracellular endopeptidases that selectively degrade components of the extracellular matrix (ECM) [84]. MMP are key enzymes for normal ECM turnover and for breakdown of ECM associated with inflammatory reactions and wound healing [110].

MMP-9, produced by macrophages, neutrophils, mast cells, eosinophils, epithelial cells, conjunctival fibroblasts, T-lymphocytes, and monocytes [84, 111], is implicated in tear destabilization and disruption of the barrier function of the ocular surface epithelium [14].

Kumagai and associates demonstrated in their study that the prevalence of active forms of MMP-2 and MMP-9 was significantly higher in patients with VKC than those with allergic conjunctivitis [112]. Although, non-allergic conjunctiva contained the proform of MMP-2 and MMP-9, the active forms of MMP-2 and MMP-9 were absent. It has been demonstrated that the marked presence of the active forms of MMP-2 and MMP-9 plays a role in the pathogenesis of corneal lesions in VKC, as well as allergic inflammation in the conjunctiva [112, 113].

Memory Cells

B- and T-lymphocytes activated by antigen differentiate into effector cells. As the immune response subsides, the majority of recently expanded effector cells are culled by apoptosis, and the effector cells that escape the culling process form the memory cells that live to mount a more rapid and efficient secondary immune response upon re-exposure to the same allergen [36]. The memory cells will readily differentiate into effector cells upon re-exposure to their specific antigen [17].

Naïve and memory T-lymphocytes express high levels of IL-7R and low levels of IL-15R. Memory T-lymphocytes express higher levels of CD44 than naïve T-lymphocytes. Naïve T-lymphocytes and central memory T-lymphocytes express CCR7 chemokine receptor, whereas effector memory T-lymphocytes expresses CCR1, CCR3 and CCR5 chemokine receptors for proinflammatory chemokines. Central memory T-lymphocytes reside in lymphoid tissue, whereas effector memory T-lymphocytes reside in non-lymphoid peripheral tissue. Effector T-lymphocytes are more readily to be triggered to proliferate and secrete cytokine, since they express high levels of IL-2R, IL-4R and IL-15R [36, 56, 114]. During the process of T-lymphocyte proliferation and differentiation, antigenic stimulation downregulates IL-7R and upregulates the expression of IL-2R and IL-15R. It is of note that IL-7 and IL-15 contributes to maintaining the pool of memory T-lymphocytes and IL-7 enhances the survival of memory T-lymphocytes through antigen-independent mechanisms [36, 65]. The high binding avidity of memory T-lymphocytes to APC could be attributed to its increased expression of accessory adhesion molecules, such as LFA-1 [36, 56]. In order to maintain long-term memory, memory cells acquired during the adaptive immune response require periodic re-stimulation with antigen and expansion of antigen-specific memory cells [36].

Neutrophils

Neutrophils are efficient phagocytes and act as important effector cells [25, 39]. Neutrophils, unlike macrophages, are short-lived immune cells that die soon after phagocytosis is completed. Neutrophils and macrophages can secrete prostaglandins, leukotrienes, and platelet activating factor [1]. Neutrophils secrete IL-1β, TNF-α, IL-6, IL-17A, IL-17F, MMP-9, neutrophil elastase, and myeloperoxidase [54]. They are the first immune cells to arrive at a site of infection, with monocytes and immature dendritic cells being recruited later [1]. Neutrophils, the most abundant and important immune cell in innate immunity, is capable of engulfing and destroying a wide range of microorganisms [17]. They play a role in T-lymphocyte mediated inflammatory reactions of the ocular surface [115]. Neutrophils and neutrophil-derived mediators (neutrophil myeloperoxidase, neutrophil elastase) are also increased in chronic ocular allergies such as VKC and AKC [116].

Platelet Activating Factor

Platelet activating factor (PAF) is a lipid mediator that plays a role in activating neutrophils, eosinophils and platelets. It also amplifies the production of lipid mediators as well as attracts leukocytes to the site of inflammation. It also amplifies the production of lipid mediators [9, 117]. Most cells involved in inflammation synthesize PAF. PAF is the most potent chemotactic agent for eosinophils [117]. Thus, it plays a major role in allergic eye diseases.

Prostaglandins

Prostaglandin is a potent inflammatory mediator formed from the cyclooxygenase pathway of arachidonic acid metabolism [25, 106]. Prostaglandin D2 (PGD2) is the major cyclooxygenase metabolite of arachidonic acid produced by mast cells in response to IgE-mediated mast cell activation. It recruits Th2-lymphocytes and eosinophils, since they express PGD2 receptor protein [9]. PGD2 acts as a mediator in allergic disorders of the eye [118]. An increase in the production of PGD2 has been observed by human mast cells via IgG1-dependent mechanisms [96]. Prostaglandins E1 (PGE1) and PGE2 produce vasodilation, redness, swelling, and pain [106].

T-Lymphocytes

T cells are lymphocytes, developed in the thymus, which have definite cell markers called TCR. T-lymphocytes initiate the immune response, mediate antigen-specific effector responses and regulate the activity of other leukocytes by secreting cytokines [16, 31]

The interaction between dendritic cells and naïve T-lymphocytes leads to the production of effector T-lymphocytes. The three key roles of the effector T-lymphocytes include killing, activation, and regulation [17, 36]. CD8+T-lymphocytes are primarily killer T-lymphocytes that recognize peptide:MHC class I complexes whereas CD4[+]T-lymphocytes are mainly helper T-lymphocytes that recognize peptide:MHC class II complexes on APC. CD8[+]T-lymphocytes differentiate into cytotoxic T-lymphocyte that destroy intracellular pathogen especially viruses [43]. Additionally, CD8[+]T-lymphocytes differentiate into Tc1-, Tc2-, Tc17-lymphocytes, regulatory CD8[+]T-lymphocytes (Tcreg), and memory (effector or central) CD8[+]T-lymphocytes [65]. CD4[+]T-lymphocytes differentiate into Th1-, Th2-, Th9-, Th17-, Th22-, Th25-lymphocytes, regulatory CD4[+]T-lymphocytes, and memory (effector or central) CD4[+]T-lymphocytes [54].

Helper T-lymphocytes provide signals to activate antigen-stimulated B-lymphocytes, macrophages and CD8[+]T-lymphocytes [17]. Th1-lymphocytes secrete IL-2, which plays a role in supporting the proliferation of CD8[+]T-lymphocytes that act as professional killers of virus-infected cells and other intracellular pathogens [36]. Additionally, Th1-lymphocytes can stimulate macrophage's microbicidal activity to enable it destroy intracellular microorganism. Th1-lymphocytes can trigger the production of antibodies (IgG1 and IgG3) against extracellular pathogens by producing co-stimulatory signals for antigen-activated naive B-lymphocytes [43].

Th2-lymphocytes provide help in B-lymphocyte activation and secrete the B-lymphocyte growth factors IL-4, IL-5, IL-9, and IL-13 that enhances B-lymphocyte proliferation and differentiation into antibody secreting cells that produce immunoglobulins, such as IgE [43]. IL-5 secreted by Th2-lymphocytes plays a crucial role in the late phase of allergic eye diseases. Th2-lymphocytes derived cytokines are responsible for the production of IgE, activation of mast cells, and recruitment and activation of eosinophils. Thus, Th2-lymphocytes play a pivotal role in the development of allergic disorders [119].

Th9-lymphocytes secrete large quantities of IL-9 and small quantities of IL-4 [120]. It also produces IL-10 [54]. Th9-lymphocytes play a role in tissue inflammation [69], as well as activate mast cells to release pro-inflammatory mediators [120]. The receptor for IL-9 is expressed on subsets of T- and B-lymphocytes, mast cells, macrophages, dendritic cells, and epithelial cells [120].

Th17-lymphocytes produce IL-17, CXCLl, CCL20, TNF-α, IL-6, IL-21, IL-22, and IL-26 [121]. It promotes acute inflammatory response by providing help in recruiting neutrophils to sites of inflammation and infection early in the adaptive immune response [43]. Allergen-specific Th17-lymphocytes can lead to secretion of IL-17, which increases eosinophilic infiltration and recruitment of macrophages to the site of allergic response [67]. Th17-lymphocyte derived cytokines (IL-17A, IL-17F, IL-21, and IL-22) trigger nonimmune cells (e.g. epithelial cells, fibroblasts, endothelial cells) to express pro-inflammatory cytokines and chemokines that induce inflammation at the site of allergic response [36]. CCL20 is a chemoattractant for neutrophils [57].

Th22-lymphocytes are skin-homing CD4$^+$T-lymphocytes that secrete IL-22 that participates in the tissue damage in chronic atopic dermatitis [54, 63]. Because of its production of IL-22 and the expression of skin homing chemokine receptors (CCR4 and CCR10), it could play a role in skin pathology [122].

Regulatory T-lymphocytes suppress the activity of other lymphocytes and help control immune responses [17]. Two main groups of regulatory T-lymphocytes are natural regulatory T-lymphocytes (Treg) and adaptive (inducible) regulatory T-lymphocytes. The natural regulatory T-lymphocytes are committed to an immunoregulatory fate while still in the thymus, whereas the adaptive variety differentiates from naïve T-lymphocytes in response to antigen [43]. Natural Tregs constitute 5-10% of CD4$^+$T-lymphocytes [36]. Regulatory T-lymphocytes downregulates allergen-induced specific T-lymphocyte activation and IgE production, as well as suppress effector cells of allergic inflammation such as mast cells and eosinophils [69]. It is of note that regulatory T-lymphocytes derived cytokines, IL-10 and TGF-β induce synthesis of noninflammatory IgG4 and IgA, respectively. Additionally, regulatory T-lymphocytes can downregulate the expression of B7 on dendritic cells [69]. Natural Tregs express high levels of CTLA-4, which inhibits T-lymphocyte activation [69].

Thymic Stromal Lymphopoietin

Epithelial cells and epidermal keratocytes express thymic stromal lymphopoietin (TSLP), an IL-7-like epithelial cell-derived pro-allergic cytokine. Furthermore, mast cells, smooth muscle cells, fibroblasts, and dendritic cells could also secrete TSLP [8]. The human TSLP gene is located on chromosome 5q22 [44]. It is noteworthy that transcription factors, nuclear factor-kappa B (NF-κB) and activator protein-1 (AP-1) contribute to TSLP gene expression [8]. TSLP can activate conventional dendritic cells to induce a Th2-lymphocyte-mediated inflammatory reaction characterized by expression of high levels of TNF-α and low levels of IL-10 [123]. TSLP primes naïve T-lymphocytes to release pro-allergic cytokines, such as IL-4, -5, and -13 [124].

Furthermore, TSLP promotes activation and differentiation of human CD8+T-lymphocytes into pro-allergic CD8$^+$T-lymphocytes [44].

Allergens in contact with epithelial cells can trigger the production of TSLP, which results in the initiation of the sensitization process and the exacerbation of allergic eye diseases [8]. TSLP activates dendritic cells to induce Th2-lymphocyte differentiation and allergic inflammation through TSLP-TSLPR (TSLP receptor chain) and OX40L-OX40 signaling pathways [125]. Thus, TSLP plays a role in the pathogenesis of severe chronic ocular allergy through the activation of dendritic cells or mast cells in synergy with proinflammatory cytokines such as IL-33 [124].

Toll-Like Receptors

Toll-like receptors (TLRs) are glycoprotein cell receptors that recognize a wide variety of exogenous and endogenous molecules, including protozoa, bacteria, and viruses [126]. TLRs are part of the body's innate immune system and it is the first-line of defense against many pathogenic and danger signals [30]. As such, it triggers the innate immune response and links innate and adaptive immunity. There are more than 10 TLRs in humans. TLRs are expressed on both non-immune (epithelial, endothelial cells) and immune cells (monocytes, APCs, lymphocytes, mast cells, neutrophils, NK cells, and eosinophils) [126, 127]. Cell-surface TLRs include TLR-1, -2, -4, -5, -6, and -10. Intracellular TLRs (TLR-3, -7, -8, and -9) recognize nucleic acids located in endosomes. TLR signaling is activated when ligands interact with adapter molecules, such as MyD88 (myeloid differentiation factor 88), MAL (MyD88 adaptor-like), TRIF (TIR domain-containing adaptor-inducing IFN-β), and TRAM (TRIP-related adaptor molecule) [1]. In MyD88-dependent pathways (all TLRs except TLR-3), the interaction between MyD88 TIR (Toll/Interleukin-1 receptor) domain and TIR domain of TLR, results in the recruitment and activation of IL1-receptor associated kinase (IRAK)-1 and -4. The activated IRAK dissociates from MyD88, and recruits TNF receptor associated factor (TRAF)-6. TRAF-6 recruits and activates TGF-β-activated protein kinase (TAK-1). Activated TAK-1 activate mitogen-activated protein kinases (MAPK) and IκB kinase (IKK) complex. Activated MAPK induces the activation of AP-1 transcription factors, whereas activated IKK phosphorylates IκB, which releases NF-κB. Translocation of NF-κB into the nucleus results in transcription of genes for pro-inflammatory cytokines, chemokines and adhesion molecules. Interaction of ligands with intracellular

TLRs except TLR-3 results in signaling through MyD88 to activate interferon regulatory factor (IRF) transcription factor that induces the production of type I interferons [1, 68, 128, 129]. The MyD88-independent pathway uses TRIF as an adaptor molecule. TRIF binds and activates inhibitor-κB kinase ε (IκKε) and TANK-binding kinase 1 (TBK1), which in turn, phosphorylates IRF37, leading to the expression of IFN-β. TLR signaling induces intracellular responses that result in the production of inflammatory cytokines, chemokines, antimicrobial peptides, and antiviral cytokines [1, 68, 130].

Pro-inflammatory mediators, proteases, and oxidative free radicals can cause inflammation and tissue injury resulting in the release of endogenous TLR ligands, known as damage-associated molecular patterns (DAMPs), which are potent inflammatory stimuli. These endogenous danger signals subsequently induce a pro-inflammatory cascade by activating TLRs, upregulating pro-inflammatory mediators and triggering further tissue damage leading to increasing levels of DAMPs [129]. DAMPs such as heat shock proteins (HSPs), hyaluronan, extra domain A of fibronectins, heparan sulfate, and fibrinogen can activate TLR2 and TLR4 [128, 129]. PAMPs (pathogen-derived ligands) are conserved structural moieties of pathogens that are detected by the innate immune sensors. Because PAMPs are produced only by microbes and not by host cells, the innate immune system is able to distinguish between self and non-self [68]. Lipoteichoic acids of Gram-positive bacteria cell walls and the lipopolysaccharide (LPS) of the outer membrane of Gram-negative bacteria are PAMPs that activate TLR on immune and non-immune cells [1].

TLR-2, TLR-4, and TLR-6 are expressed on mast cells, and activation of TLR-2 and TLR-4 can induce mast cell degranulation and release of Th2-lymphocyte cytokines [126]. An increased expression and activation of TLR4 in chronic allergic keratoconjunctivitis may lead to overproduction of proinflammatory cytokines and chemokines, which may exacerbate the ongoing inflammatory response. TLR2-mediated cytokine and chemokine production may exacerbate the inflammatory response in patients with AKC [127]. TSLP initiates the development of ocular allergy via TLR-mediated innate response in epithelial cells. Because TLR4 responds to DAMP, it is likely that pollen could serve as a functional TLR4 agonist that induces expression of TSLP via TLR and NF-κB signaling to trigger Th2-lymphocyte-mediated allergic ocular surface inflammation [131, 132]. Therefore, TLRs play a vital role in the ocular surface immune response [30], as TLR in the corneal and conjunctival epithelium is activated during ocular allergic conditions [133].

References

[1] Murphy, K.P., Travers, P., Walport, M., The Induced Response of Innate Immunity, in *Janeway's Immunobiology*. 2012, Garland Science: New York. p. 75-125.

[2] Irkeç, M. and B. Bozkurt, Epithelial cells in ocular allergy. *Curr Allergy Asthma Rep*, 2003. 3(4): p. 352-7.

[3] Langer, H.F. and T. Chavakis, Leukocyte-endothelial interactions in inflammation. *J Cell Mol Med*, 2009. 13(7): p. 1211-20.

[4] Abu el-Asrar, A., et al., Adhesion molecules in vernal keratoconjunctivitis. *Br J Ophthalmol*, 1997. 81(12): p. 1099-106.

[5] Carlos, T.M. and J.M. Harlan, Leukocyte-endothelial adhesion molecules. *Blood*, 1994. 84(7): p. 2068-101.

[6] Zhan, H., et al., Clinical and immunological features of atopic keratoconjunctivitis. *Int Ophthalmol Clin*, 2003. 43(1): p. 59-71.

[7] Lalor, P.F., et al., Vascular adhesion protein-1 mediates adhesion and transmigration of lymphocytes on human hepatic endothelial cells. *J Immunol*, 2002. 169(2): p. 983-92.

[8] Takai, T., TSLP expression: cellular sources, triggers, and regulatory mechanisms. *Allergol Int*, 2012. 61(1): p. 3-17.

[9] Murphy, K.P., Travers, P., Walport, M., Allergy and Allergic Diseases, in *Janeway's Immunobiology*. 2012, Garland Science: New York. p. 571-610.

[10] Matsumura, Y., Role of Allergen Source-Derived Proteases in Sensitization via Airway Epithelial Cells. *J Allergy* (Cairo), 2012. 2012: p. 903659.

[11] Takai, T. and S. Ikeda, Barrier dysfunction caused by environmental proteases in the pathogenesis of allergic diseases. *Allergol Int*, 2011. 60(1): p. 25-35.

[12] Ohbayashi, M., et al., The Role of Histamine in Ocular Allergy. *Adv Exp Med Biol*, 2010. 709: p. 43-52.

[13] Delves, P., et al., Allergy and Other hypersensitivities, in Roitt's Essential Immunology. 2011, *Wiley-Blackwell*. p. 394-422.

[14] Stern, M.E., et al., Autoimmunity at the ocular surface: pathogenesis and regulation. *Mucosal Immunol*, 2010. 3(5): p. 425-42.

[15] Male, D.C., Anne; Owen, Michael; Trowsdale, John; Champion, Brian. , B cell Activation and Maturation. *Advanced Immunology*. 1996: Mosby Co. 9.1-9.16.

[16]   Chigbu, D.I., The pathophysiology of ocular allergy: a review. *Cont Lens Anterior Eye,* 2009. 32(1): p. 3-15; quiz 43-4.

[17]   Murphy, K.P., Travers, P., Walport, M., Basic Concepts in Immunology, in Janeway's Immunobiology. 2012, *Garland Science:* New York. p. 1-36.

[18]   Murphy, K.P., Travers, P., Walport, M., The Humoral Immune Response, in Janeway's Immunobiology. 2012, *Garland Science:* New York. p. 387-428.

[19]   Knop, N. and E. Knop, Conjunctiva-associated lymphoid tissue in the human eye. *Invest Ophthalmol Vis Sci,* 2000. 41(6): p. 1270-9.

[20]   Knop, E. and N. Knop, Anatomy and immunology of the ocular surface. *Chem Immunol Allergy,* 2007. 92: p. 36-49.

[21]   Delves, P., et al., Antibodies, in Roitt's Essential Immunology. 2011, *Wiley-Blackwell.* p. 53-78.

[22]   Adkinson, N.F.J., The Basic Immunology of Allergic Diseases. *Allergy Proc,* 1990. 11(1): p. 5-6.

[23]   Delves, P., et al., Lymphocyte Activation, in Roitt's Essential Immunology. 2011, *Wiley-Blackwell.* p. 205-225.

[24]   Trinh, L., et al., Th1 and Th2 responses on the ocular surface in uveitis identified by CCR4 and CCR5 conjunctival expression. *Am J Ophthalmol,* 2007. 144(4): p. 580-5.

[25]   Cousins, S.W. and B.T. Rouse, Chemical Mediators of Ocular Inflammation In: Pepose JS, Holland GN, Wilhelmus KR, editors. *Ocular Infection and Immunity.* 1996, St Louis: Mosby. 50-70.

[26]   Revillard, J., Innate immunity. *Eur J Dermatol.* 12(3): p. 224-7.

[27]   Turner, M., Molecules which recognize Antigen. In: Roitt I, Brostoff J and Male D, editors. *Immunology.* 1989, St. Louis: The C.V. Mosby Co. 5.1-5.12.

[28]   Murphy, K.P., Travers, P., Walport, M., Signalimg Through Immune-System Receptors, in Janeway's Immunobiology. 2012, *Garland Science:* New York. p. 239-274.

[29]   Male, D.C., Anne; Owen, Michael; Trowsdale, John; Champion, Brian. , Antigen Processing and Presentation. *Advanced Immunology.* 1996: Mosby Co. 7.1-7.20.

[30]   Gilger, B.C., Immunology of the ocular surface. *Vet Clin North Am Small Anim Pract,* 2008. 38(2): p. 223-31, v.

[31]   Lanier, L., Cells of the Immune Response: Lymphocytes and Mononuclear Phagocytes. In: Stites DP, Terr AI, editors. Basic Human

Immunology., ed. D.P. Stites and A.I. Terr. 1991, Norwalk, Connecticut: Appleton and Lange. 61-72.

[32]   Male, D., Introduction to the Immune System. In: Male D, Brostoff J, Roth DB, Roitt I, editors. Immunology. . 2006.: *Mosby Elsevier.* 3-18

[33]   Lund, F.E., Cytokine-producing B lymphocytes-key regulators of immunity. *Curr Opin Immunol,* 2008. 20(3): p. 332-8.

[34]   Mauri, C. and A. Bosma, Immune regulatory function of B cells. *Annu Rev Immunol,* 2012. 30: p. 221-41.

[35]   Noh, G. and J.H. Lee, Regulatory B cells and allergic diseases. *Allergy Asthma Immunol Res,* 2011. 3(3): p. 168-77.

[36]   Delves, P., et al., The Production of Effectors in Roitt's Essential Immunology. 2011, *Wiley-Blackwell.* p. 226-262.

[37]   Leonardi, A. and A. Secchi, Vernal keratoconjunctivitis. *Int Ophthalmol Clin,* 2003. 43(1): p. 41-58.

[38]   Murphy, K.P., Travers, P., Walport, M., Innate Immunity: The First Lines of Defense, in Janeway's Immunobiology. 2012, *Garland Science:* New York. p. 37-74.

[39]   Delves, P., et al., Innate Immunity, in Roitt's Essential Immunology. 2011, *Wiley-Blackwell.* p. 3-34.

[40]   Leonardi, A., C. De Dominicis, and L. Motterle, Immunopathogenesis of ocular allergy: a schematic approach to different clinical entities. *Curr Opin Allergy Clin Immunol,* 2007. 7(5): p. 429-35.

[41]   Murphy, K.P.T., Paul; Walport, Mark; Janeway, Charles T-cell mediated immunity. Janeway's immunobiology 7th ed. 2008, New York *Garland Science* 323-378.

[42]   Murphy, K.T., Paul; Walport, Mark; Janeway, Charles Signaling through immune system receptors. Janeway's Immunobiology. 7th ed. 2008, New York: *Garland Science.* 219-256.

[43]   Murphy, K.P., Travers, P., Walport, M., T Cell-Mediated Immunity, in Janeway's Immunobiology. 2012, *Garland Science:* New York. p. 335-386.

[44]   He, R. and R.S. Geha, Thymic stromal lymphopoietin. *Ann N Y Acad Sci,* 2010. 1183: p. 13-24.

[45]   Jenkins, S.J., et al., Dendritic cell expression of OX40 ligand acts as a costimulatory, not polarizing, signal for optimal Th2 priming and memory induction in vivo. *J Immunol,* 2007. 179(6): p. 3515-23.

[46]   Wilson, S.E. and A. Esposito, Focus on molecules: interleukin-1: a master regulator of the corneal response to injury. *Exp Eye Res,* 2009. 89(2): p. 124-5.

[47]   Asano-Kato, N., et al., TGF-beta1, IL-1beta, and Th2 cytokines stimulate vascular endothelial growth factor production from conjunctival fibroblasts. *Exp Eye Res,* 2005. 80(4): p. 555-60.

[48]   Zhang, L., et al., Increased frequencies of Th22 cells as well as Th17 cells in the peripheral blood of patients with ankylosing spondylitis and rheumatoid arthritis. *PLoS One,* 2012. 7(4): p. e31000.

[49]   Ozcan, A., T. Ersoz, and E. Dulger, Management of severe allergic conjunctivitis with topical cyclosporin a 0.05% eyedrops. *Cornea,* 2007. 26(9): p. 1035-8.

[50]   Solomon, A., I. Puxeddu, and F. Levi-Schaffer, Fibrosis in ocular allergic inflammation: recent concepts in the pathogenesis of ocular allergy. *Curr Opin Allergy Clin Immunol,* 2003. 3(5): p. 389-93.

[51]   Uchio, E., et al., Tear levels of interferon-gamma, interleukin (IL) -2, IL-4 and IL-5 in patients with vernal keratoconjunctivitis, atopic keratoconjunctivitis and allergic conjunctivitis. *Clin Exp Allergy,* 2000. 30(1): p. 103-9.

[52]   Soroosh, P. and T.A. Doherty, Th9 and allergic disease. *Immunology,* 2009. 127(4): p. 450-8.

[53]   Stassen, M., E. Schmitt, and T. Bopp, From interleukin-9 to T helper 9 cells. *Ann N Y Acad Sci,* 2012. 1247: p. 56-68.

[54]   Vock, C., H.P. Hauber, and M. Wegmann, The other T helper cells in asthma pathogenesis. *J Allergy* (Cairo), 2010. 2010: p. 519298.

[55]   Li, J., R.C. Tripathi, and B.J. Tripathi, Drug-induced ocular disorders. *Drug Saf,* 2008. 31(2): p. 127-41.

[56]   Murphy, K.P., Travers, P., Walport, M., Dynamics of Adaptive Immunity, in Janeway's Immunobiology. 2012, *Garland Science:* New York. p. 429-464.

[57]   Tesmer, L.A., et al., Th17 cells in human disease. *Immunol Rev,* 2008. 223: p. 87-113.

[58]   Guglani, L. and S.A. Khader, Th17 cytokines in mucosal immunity and inflammation. *Curr Opin HIV AIDS,* 2010. 5(2): p. 120-7.

[59]   Ma, P., et al., Human corneal epithelium-derived thymic stromal lymphopoietin links the innate and adaptive immune responses via TLRs and Th2 cytokines. *Invest Ophthalmol Vis Sci,* 2009. 50(6): p. 2702-9.

[60]   Ouyang, W., J.K. Kolls, and Y. Zheng, The biological functions of T helper 17 cell effector cytokines in inflammation. *Immunity,* 2008. 28(4): p. 454-67.

[61]   Sarra, M., et al., Interleukin-21 in immune and allergic diseases. *Inflamm Allergy Drug Targets,* 2012. 11(4): p. 313-9.

[62] Cavani, A., D. Pennino, and K. Eyerich, Th17 and Th22 in skin allergy. *Chem Immunol Allergy,* 2012. 96: p. 39-44.

[63] Souwer, Y., et al., IL-17 and IL-22 in atopic allergic disease. *Curr Opin Immunol,* 2010. 22(6): p. 821-6.

[64] Miller, A.M., Role of IL-33 in inflammation and disease. *J Inflamm* (Lond), 2011. 8(1): p. 22.

[65] Shrikant, P.A., et al., Regulating functional cell fates in CD8 T cells. *Immunol Res,* 2010. 46(1-3): p. 12-22.

[66] Chen, W., Dendritic cells and (CD4+)CD25+ T regulatory cells: crosstalk between two professionals in immunity versus tolerance. *Front Biosci,* 2006. 11: p. 1360-70.

[67] Akkoc, T., M. Akdis, and C.A. Akdis, Update in the mechanisms of allergen-specific immunotheraphy. *Allergy Asthma Immunol Res,* 2011. 3(1): p. 11-20.

[68] Kumar, A. and F.S. Yu, Toll-like receptors and corneal innate immunity. *Curr Mol Med,* 2006. 6(3): p. 327-37.

[69] Jutel, M. and C.A. Akdis, T-cell subset regulation in atopy. *Curr Allergy Asthma Rep,* 2011. 11(2): p. 139-45.

[70] Blasius, A.L. and B. Beutler, Intracellular toll-like receptors. *Immunity,* 2010. 32(3): p. 305-15.

[71] Spencer, L.A. and P.F. Weller, Eosinophils and Th2 immunity: contemporary insights. *Immunol Cell Biol,* 2010. 88(3): p. 250-6.

[72] Shi, H.Z., Eosinophils function as antigen-presenting cells. *J Leukoc Biol,* 2004. 76(3): p. 520-7.

[73] Abu El-Asrar, A., et al., Expression of chemokine receptors in vernal keratoconjunctivitis. *Br J Ophthalmol,* 2001. 85(11): p. 1357-61.

[74] Abu El-Asrar, A., et al., Chemokines in the limbal form of vernal keratoconjunctivitis. *Br J Ophthalmol,* 2000. 84(12): p. 1360-6.

[75] Kimura, K., S. Teranishi, and T. Nishida, Interleukin-1beta-induced disruption of barrier function in cultured human corneal epithelial cells. *Invest Ophthalmol Vis Sci,* 2009. 50(2): p. 597-603.

[76] Calonge, M. and A. Enríquez-de-Salamanca, The role of the conjunctival epithelium in ocular allergy. *Curr Opin Allergy Clin Immunol,* 2005. 5(5): p. 441-5.

[77] Hingorani, M., et al., The role of conjunctival epithelial cells in chronic ocular allergic disease. *Exp Eye Res,* 1998. 67(5): p. 491-500.

[78] Iwata, M., et al., CD40 expression in normal human cornea and regulation of CD40 in cultured human corneal epithelial and stromal cells. *Invest Ophthalmol Vis Sci,* 2002. 43(2): p. 348-57.

[79] Xi, X., et al., Ocular fibroblast diversity: implications for inflammation and ocular wound healing. *Invest Ophthalmol Vis Sci*, 2011. 52(7): p. 4859-65.

[80] Kumagai, N., et al., Role of structural cells of the cornea and conjunctiva in the pathogenesis of vernal keratoconjunctivitis. *Prog Retin Eye Res,* 2006. 25(2): p. 165-87.

[81] Fukuda, K., et al., Fibroblasts as local immune modulators in ocular allergic disease. *Allergol Int,* 2006. 55(2): p. 121-9.

[82] Enriquez-de-Salamanca, A., et al., Tear cytokine and chemokine analysis and clinical correlations in evaporative-type dry eye disease. *Mol Vis,* 2010. 16: p. 862-73.

[83] Lambiase, A., et al., Expression of nerve growth factor receptors on the ocular surface in healthy subjects and during manifestation of inflammatory diseases. *Invest Ophthalmol Vis Sci,* 1998. 39(7): p. 1272-5.

[84] Kumar, S., Vernal keratoconjunctivitis: a major review. *Acta Ophthalmol,* 2009. 87(2): p. 133-47.

[85] Leonardi, A., et al., Transforming growth factor-beta/Smad - signalling pathway and conjunctival remodelling in vernal keratoconjunctivitis. *Clin Exp Allergy,* 2011. 41(1): p. 52-60.

[86] Leonardi, A., L. Motterle, and M. Bortolotti, Allergy and the eye. *Clin Exp Immunol,* 2008. 153 Suppl 1: p. 17-21.

[87] Lambiase, A., et al., Increased plasma levels of nerve growth factor in vernal keratoconjunctivitis and relationship to conjunctival mast cells. *Invest Ophthalmol Vis Sci,* 1995. 36(10): p. 2127-32.

[88] Jacob, S.E. and M.P. Castanedo-Tardan, Pharmacotherapy for allergic contact dermatitis. *Expert Opin Pharmacother,* 2007. 8(16): p. 2757-74.

[89] Bielory, L. and S. Ghafoor, Histamine receptors and the conjunctiva. *Curr Opin Allergy Clin Immunol,* 2005. 5(5): p. 437-40.

[90] Nakano, Y., et al., Role of histamine H(4) receptor in allergic conjunctivitis in mice. *Eur J Pharmacol,* 2009. 608(1-3): p. 71-5.

[91] Tabbara, K., Immunopathogenesis of chronic allergic conjunctivitis. *Int Ophthalmol Clin,* 2003. 43(1): p. 1-7.

[92] Deschenes, J., M. Discepola, and M. Abelson, Comparative evaluation of olopatadine ophthalmic solution (0.1%) versus ketorolac ophthalmic solution (0.5%) using the provocative antigen challenge model. *Acta Ophthalmol Scand Suppl,* 1999(228): p. 47-52.

[93] Beltrani, V.S. and V.P. Beltrani, Contact dermatitis. *Ann Allergy Asthma Immunol,* 1997. 78(2): p. 160-73; quiz 174-6.

[94] Abu-El-Asrar, A., et al., Langerhans' cells in vernal keratoconjunctivitis express the costimulatory molecule B7-2 (CD86), but not B7-1 (CD80). *Eye*, 2001. 15(Pt 5): p. 648-54.

[95] Terr, A.I., Inflammation. In: Stites DP, Terr AI, Parslow TG, editors. Medical Immunology. 1997, Stamford, Connecticut: Appleton and Lange. 182-195.

[96] Woolhiser, M., et al., IgG-dependent activation of human mast cells following up-regulation of FcgammaRI by IFN-gamma. *Eur J Immunol*, 2001. 31(11): p. 3298-307.

[97] Bielory, L., et al., Treating the ocular component of allergic rhinoconjunctivitis and related eye disorders. *MedGenMed*, 2007. 9(3): p. 35.

[98] Elhers, W. and P. Donshik, Giant papillary conjunctivitis. *Curr Opin Allergy Clin Immunol*, 2008. 8(5): p. 445-9.

[99] Bonini, S., et al., Vernal keratoconjunctivitis. *Eye*, 2004. 18(4): p. 345-51.

[100] Owen, M., Major Histocompatibility Complex. In: Roitt I, Brostoff J and Male D, editors. *Immunology.*, ed. B.J.M.D. Roitt I. 1989, St. Louis: The C.V. *Mosby* Co. 4.1-4.12.

[101] Murphy, K.P., Travers, P., Walport, M., Antigen Presentation to T-Lymphocytes, in Janeway's Immunobiology. 2012, *Garland Science:* New York. p. 201-237.

[102] Murphy, K.P., Travers, P., Walport, M., Antigen Recognition by B-cell and T-cell Receptors, in Janeway's Immunobiology. 2012, *Garland Science:* New York. p. 127-156.

[103] Irani, A.M., Ocular mast cells and mediators. *Immunol Allergy Clin North Am*, 2008. 28(1): p. 25-42, v.

[104] Malbec, O. and M. Daëron, The mast cell IgG receptors and their roles in tissue inflammation. *Immunol Rev*, 2007. 217: p. 206-21.

[105] Leonardi, A., Pathophysiology of allergic conjunctivitis. *Acta Ophthalmol Scand Suppl*, 1999(228): p. 21-3.

[106] Howarth, P., Antihistamines in rhinoconjunctivitis. *Clin Allergy Immunol*, 2002. 17: p. 179-220.

[107] Leonardi, A., The central role of conjunctival mast cells in the pathogenesis of ocular allergy. *Curr Allergy Asthma Rep*, 2002. 2(4): p. 325-31.

[108] Brown, J., T. Wilson, and D. Metcalfe, The mast cell and allergic diseases: role in pathogenesis and implications for therapy. *Clin Exp Allergy*, 2008. 38(1): p. 4-18.

[109] Schafermeyer, R.W., et al., Respiratory effects of spinal immobilization in children. *Ann Emerg Med,* 1991. 20(9): p. 1017-9.

[110] Abu El-Asrar, A., et al., Gelatinase B in vernal keratoconjunctivitis. *Arch Ophthalmol,* 2001. 119(10): p. 1505-11.

[111] Leonardi, A., et al., Matrix metalloproteases in vernal keratoconjunctivitis, nasal polyps and allergic asthma. *Clin Exp Allergy,* 2007. 37(6): p. 872-9.

[112] Kumagai, N., et al., Active matrix metalloproteinases in the tear fluid of individuals with vernal keratoconjunctivitis. *J Allergy Clin Immunol,* 2002. 110(3): p. 489-91.

[113] Tuft, S.J., et al., Limbal vernal keratoconjunctivitis in the tropics. *Ophthalmology,* 1998. 105(8): p. 1489-93.

[114] Cui, W. and S.M. Kaech, Generation of effector CD8+ T cells and their conversion to memory T cells. *Immunol Rev,* 2010. 236: p. 151-66.

[115] Shimmura, S., et al., Lecithin-bound superoxide dismutase in the treatment of noninfectious corneal ulcers. *Am J Ophthalmol,* 2003. 135(5): p. 613-9.

[116] Cook, E.B., Tear cytokines in acute and chronic ocular allergic inflammation. *Curr Opin Allergy Clin Immunol,* 2004. 4(5): p. 441-5.

[117] Zinchuk, O., et al., Direct action of platelet activating factor (PAF) induces eosinophil accumulation and enhances expression of PAF receptors in conjunctivitis. *Mol Vis,* 2005. 11: p. 114-23.

[118] Fujishima, H., et al., Prostaglandin D2 induces chemotaxis in eosinophils via its receptor CRTH2 and eosinophils may cause severe ocular inflammation in patients with allergic conjunctivitis. *Cornea,* 2005. 24(8 Suppl): p. S66-S70.

[119] Leonardi, A., et al., Th1- and Th2-type cytokines in chronic ocular allergy. *Graefes Arch Clin Exp Ophthalmol,* 2006. 244(10): p. 1240-5.

[120] Jager, A. and V.K. Kuchroo, Effector and regulatory T-cell subsets in autoimmunity and tissue inflammation. *Scand J Immunol,* 2010. 72(3): p. 173-84.

[121] Di Cesare, A., P. Di Meglio, and F.O. Nestle, The IL-23/Th17 axis in the immunopathogenesis of psoriasis. *J Invest Dermatol,* 2009. 129(6): p. 1339-50.

[122] Annunziato, F. and S. Romagnani, Heterogeneity of human effector CD4+ T cells. *Arthritis Res Ther,* 2009. 11(6): p. 257.

[123] Liu, Y.J., Thymic stromal lymphopoietin and OX40 ligand pathway in the initiation of dendritic cell-mediated allergic inflammation. *J Allergy Clin Immunol,* 2007. 120(2): p. 238-44; quiz 245-6.

[124] Matsuda, A., et al., Functional role of thymic stromal lymphopoietin in chronic allergic keratoconjunctivitis. *Invest Ophthalmol Vis Sci,* 2010. 51(1): p. 151-5.

[125] Zheng, X., et al., TSLP and downstream molecules in experimental mouse allergic conjunctivitis. *Invest Ophthalmol Vis Sci,* 2010. 51(6): p. 3076-82.

[126] Bonini, S., et al., Expression of Toll-like receptors in healthy and allergic conjunctiva. *Ophthalmology,* 2005. 112(9): p. 1528; discussion 1548-9.

[127] Redfern, R.L. and A.M. McDermott, Toll-like receptors in ocular surface disease. *Exp Eye Res,* 2010. 90(6): p. 679-87.

[128] Takeda, K. and S. Akira, Toll-like receptors in innate immunity. *Int Immunol,* 2005. 17(1): p. 1-14.

[129] Prince, L.R., et al., The role of TLRs in neutrophil activation. *Curr Opin Pharmacol,* 2011. 11(4): p. 397-403.

[130] Johnson, A.C., et al., Activation of toll-like receptor (TLR)2, TLR4, and TLR9 in the mammalian cornea induces MyD88-dependent corneal inflammation. *Invest Ophthalmol Vis Sci,* 2005. 46(2): p. 589-95.

[131] Li, D.Q., et al., Short ragweed pollen triggers allergic inflammation through Toll-like receptor 4-dependent thymic stromal lymphopoietin/OX40 ligand/OX40 signaling pathways. *J Allergy Clin Immunol,* 2011. 128(6): p. 1318-1325 e2.

[132] Li, D., et al., Recent Advances in Mucosal Immunology and Ocular Surface Diseases, in Advances in Ophthalmology, S. Rumelt, Editor 2012. p. 49-78.

[133] Micera, A., et al., Toll-like receptors and the eye. *Curr Opin Allergy Clin Immunol,* 2005. 5(5): p. 451-8.

Chapter 4

Immunology Relevant to Allergic Ocular Surface Diseases

The main function of the response mounted by the immune system is to discriminate between self and non-self agents and thereby eliminate what it considers to be foreign. The three levels of immune defense against invasion by foreign agents are anatomical and physicochemical barrier, active innate immunity (antigen-non-specific defense mechanism) and adaptive immunity (antigen-specific defense mechanism) [1].

The innate immunity is present from birth and provides an immediate, relatively broad response to foreign substances. The principal components of the innate immune system include cellular and humoral elements, each of which is endowed with afferent and efferent arms. The cellular components of innate immunity include macrophages, neutrophils, dendritic cells, eosinophils and mast cells. Pattern recognition receptors (PRR) are components of the afferent arm of the innate immune system involved in the detection of molecular patterns associated with pathogens or damaged host tissues. Proteases, lipases, cell adhesion molecules, and free radicals are cellular components of the efferent arm of the innate immune system. Humoral components of the innate immune system include antimicrobial peptides, lysozyme, complement, and lactoferrin [2]. The innate immune system utilizes soluble- or cell-associated PRRs to detect foreign substances that have breached the host's anatomic barriers. Once these foreign substances are detected, the immune system mounts an immediate attack, which involves attacking the foreign agents with destructive enzymes, such as proteolytic enzymes. If this process fails to remove the foreign agent within the first four hours (immediate innate stage), an early-induced innate response lasting up to four days is initiated. The recruitment and activation of effector components (neutrophils, monocytes, macrophages, mast cells, eosinophils, natural killer (NK) cells, complement, lysozyme, cytokines, chemokines, and adhesion molecules), as well as recognition of pathogen-associated molecular patterns (PAMPs) and damage-associated molecular patterns (DAMPs) characterize the early-induced innate immune response [1].

Innate immunity relies on PRR expressed on immune cells (e.g. neutrophils, macrophages, dendritic cells, monocytes) and non-immune cells (e.g. epithelial cells) to recognize PAMP (pathogen-derived ligands) and DAMP [3]. Toll-like receptors (TLR), nucleotide binding oligomerization domain (NOD)-like receptors (NLR), and RIG-I-like receptors (RLR) are PRR that act as innate immune sensors to enhance adaptive immune responses. TLR is a major innate immune receptor that can induce ocular surface APCs to produce cytokines that favor the development of allergic ocular surface diseases [4]. TLRs provide a crucial first step in the innate immune response and influence the development of adaptive immunity by activating APCs [5]. TLR-mediated activation of DCs induces DC maturation, with the production of pro-inflammatory cytokines, upregulation of co-stimulatory and major histocompatibility complex (MHC) molecules, and as such, it enhances the antigen presenting capacity of DCs. Thus, TLR stimulation of APCs leads to the activation and priming of antigen specific naive T-lymphocytes, triggering the adaptive arm of the immune response [6]. If the innate immune response is unable to remove the foreign agent, the antigen presenting cells (APC) will transport the foreign agent in a form that will be recognized by naïve T-lymphocytes within the regional lymph nodes. This will induce the proliferation and differentiation of the naïve T-lymphocytes into effector cells capable of removing the foreign agent (adaptive immune response). It takes four to five days for a functional adaptive immune response to develop [1, 7]. The adaptive immune response is composed of humoral immunity mediated by B-lymphocytes and cell-mediated immunity mediated by T-lymphocytes. Adaptive (acquired) immunity is designed to react with and remove specific antigens. It improves upon repeated exposure to a given antigen. It involves APCs; activation and proliferation of lymphocytes; differentiation of lymphocytes into effector cells and memory cells; and the production of cytokines, chemokines, and cell adhesion molecules [8-11].

Lymphocyte Activation

The CD4+T- and CD8+T-lymphocytes are involved in the pathomechanism of allergic disorders of the ocular surface. However, this chapter will focus on the activation of naïve CD4+T-lymphocytes with particular emphasis on activation, proliferation and differentiation signals. The first (activation) signal is triggered by recognition of peptide-major histocompatibility complex (MHC) by T-lymphocyte Antigen Receptor (TCR) on naïve T-lymphocyte. The second (co-stimulatory) signal involves co-stimulatory interactions. The third (differentiation) signals involve directing T-lymphocyte differentiation [12, 13]

Antigen-presenting cells (APC), such as dendritic cells, capture and process antigen into peptide fragments, which are presented as peptides in association with major histocompatibility complex (MHC) class II molecules on the surface of the APC. This results in the formation of peptide-MHC class II complex on the APC. The interaction between the TCR on naïve T-lymphocyte and peptide-MHC class II complex triggers the recruitment of coreceptors for MHC into the complex that act to enhance the ability of the naïve T-lymphocyte to respond effectively to the antigen. It is of note that CD4 molecules act as coreceptors for MHC class II and CD8 molecules act as coreceptors for MHC class I molecules [12, 14]. Thus, the complex formed between TCR and peptide-MHC class II complex provides the activation signal (signal 1) through the T-cell receptor complex (composed of TCR and CD3 coreceptor complex), and this is enhanced by coupling of CD4 molecule with the MHC class II molecule to yield CD4+T-lymphocytes. It should be noted that the interaction between TCR on naïve T-lymphocyte and peptide-MHC class I complex along with coupling of CD8 molecule to MHC class I molecule will yield CD8+T-lymphocytes. A stable association between CD4+T-lymphocytes and APCs is achieved by non-specific binding through adhesion molecules, such as ICAM-1 on the APC and LFA-1 on CD4+T-lymphocytes [12]. When peptide-MHC complex engages TCR, Src-family kinase phosphorylates immunoreceptor tyrosine-based activation motifs (ITAMs) in the TCR complex. The phosphorylated ITAMs create a binding site for recruitment and activation of ZAP-70 kinase (zeta chain-associated protein of 70 kDA) into the TCR signaling complex. The activated ZAP-70 kinase recruits and phosphorylates LAT (linker of activated T cells) and SLP-76 (SH2-domain containing leukocyte protein of 76 kDA). LAT and SLP76 recruit phospholipase Cγ (PLCγ) into the TCR complex [12, 15-17]. To achieve full CD4+T-lymphocyte activation, interaction between co-stimulatory molecule B7 (B7.1 (CD80) or B7.2 (CD86)) on the APC and co-stimulatory receptor CD28 on the CD4+T-lymphocytes is necessary (co-stimulatory or signal 2) [12]. This co-stimulatory signal is involved in promoting the survival and proliferation of naïve T-lymphocytes. Phosphorylation of PLCγ by Tec-family kinase (Itk expressed in T-lymphocytes) along with co-stimulatory signals emanating from TCR and CD28, results in the activation of PLCγ, a key signaling protein that initiates three signaling pathways that culminate in the activation of transcription factors in the nucleus [15-17]. Following activation of PLCγ, PLCγ cleaves phosphatidylinositol bisphosphate (PIP_2) to yield diacylglycerol (DAG) and inositol trisphosphate (IP_3) [12, 15-17]. Interaction of IP_3 with specific receptors (IP_3 receptors) triggers an increase in intracellular calcium concentration. Calcium interacts with calmodulin to form a calcium-calmodulin complex that binds to calcineurin, a phosphatase that dephosphorylates NFAT (nuclear factor of activated T cells). The dephosphorylation of NFAT facilitates the translocation of NFAT into the nucleus, where it binds to the IL-2 enhancer to activate the transcription genes for IL-2 production [12, 16, 18]. DAG plays an important role in the Ras-MAP kinase-signaling pathway that results in the production of the transcription factor, AP-1 (activator protein 1). Additionally, DAG activates protein kinase C θ, which in turn phosphorylate CARMA1. The phosphorylated CARMA1 activates the transcription factor, NF-κB. The transcription factors initiate gene transcription that results in the expression of cytokines that are involved in the differentiation of effector cells [12, 15-17]. Furthermore, the antigen-induced signaling pathway alters the gene expression in the nucleus leading to the synthesis of chemokines and adhesion molecules, as well as inducing the proliferation and differentiation of antigen-stimulated T-lymphocyte [17]. It is of note that transcription of IL-2 is one of the key events that prevents the signaled T-lymphocyte from lapsing into anergy [12]. The IL-2 will induce proliferation of the activated T-lymphocyte. IL-2- driven clonal expansion is followed by differentiation of the activated T-lymphocytes into antigen-specific effector T-lymphocytes and memory T-lymphocytes [13].

The activated CD4⁺T-lymphocyte proliferate into identical CD4⁺T-lymphocytes, and further differentiate into Th1-, Th2-, Th9-, Th17-, Th22-, or adaptive regulatory T-lymphocytes, as well as memory CD4⁺T-lymphocytes (signal 3 or differentiation signal) (figure 1a) [19-21]. The differentiation of CD4⁺T lymphocytes into Th1-lymphocytes is initiated by the phosphorylation of signal transducer and activator of transcription (STAT)-1 in CD4⁺ T lymphocytes by IFNγ. The phosphorylated STAT1 induces expression of T-box expressed in T cells (T-bet), which in turn switches on the IFN-γ gene in the T-lymphocyte and upregulates the expression of specific subunit of the receptor for IL-12 (IL-12Rβ2) [21, 22]. IL-12 produced by activated dendritic cells interact with IL-12Rβ2 expressed on the CD4$^+$T-lymphocytes, via a signaling pathway that activates STAT4, to promote further expansion and differentiation of the committed Th1-lymphocytes, as well as induce high production of IFN-γ [13, 21, 22]. Th1-derived cytokines promote macrophage activation; antibody-dependent cell-mediated cytotoxicity; and Th1-mediated delayed-type hypersensitivity (DTH).

The differentiation of CD4$^+$T lymphocytes into Th2-lymphocytes occurs when IL-4 produced by activated dendritic cells interacts with IL-4 receptor, which in turn results in the phosphorylation of STAT6, a transcription regulator [21, 22]. The phosphorylated STAT6 upregulates the expression of the Th2-lymphocyte transcription factor GATA-binding protein-3 (GATA-3) in CD4$^+$T lymphocytes. GATA-3 is a powerful activator of the genes for Th2-lymphocyte derived cytokines [13]. GATA3 induces the differentiation of CD4$^+$T-lymphocytes into Th2-lymphocytes, as well as transactivates Th2-specific cytokines such as IL-4, IL-5, and IL-13 [21, 22]. It is of note that Th1 and Th2 lymphocytes express the T-bet and GATA-3 transcription factors, respectively [13]. Th2-lymphocytes release cytokines that are responsible for mucosal immunity, eosinophil accumulation, IgE production, mast cells growth, and mucus hyperproduction [23-26]. Th2-like cytokines play an important pathophysiological role in ocular allergic conditions [27].

The transcription factors that are essential for Th9-lymphocyte generation are PU.1 and interferon-regulatory factor 4 (IRF4) [28]. The interaction of IL-4 and TGF-β (produced by activated dendritic cells) with their respective receptors induces signals that activate STAT6, which in turn induces the expression of PU.1 and IRF4 on the CD4$^+$T-lymphocyte. These transcription factors will initiate gene Il9 expression and differentiation of CD4$^+$T-lymphocyte into Th9-lymphocytes that secrete IL-9 [29]. IL-9 stimulates epithelial cells to release chemokines; promotes proliferation of mast cells and release of mast cell cytokines; stimulates B-lymphocytes to produce IgE and IgG; promotes eosinophil maturation and survival; and synergizes with IL-17 to promote neutrophilia at the site of allergic inflammation [30].

The differentiation of CD4+T lymphocytes into Th17-lymphocytes involves IL-6 (IL-6 produced by dendritic cells) signaling in the presence of TGF-β leading to phosphorylation of STAT3, which in turn induces the expression of retinoic acid-related orphan receptor (ROR)γt/ RORα in CD4$^+$T-lymphocytes. The generated RORγT/RORα triggers the differentiation of

CD4+T-lymphocytes into Th17-lymphocytes that secrete IL-17A, IL-17F, IL-22, and IL-26 [13, 22, 31]. IL-17A and IL-17F induces epithelial cells, fibroblast and endothelial cells to secrete cytokines and chemokines that induce chronic neutrophilia at the site of inflammation [13, 32].

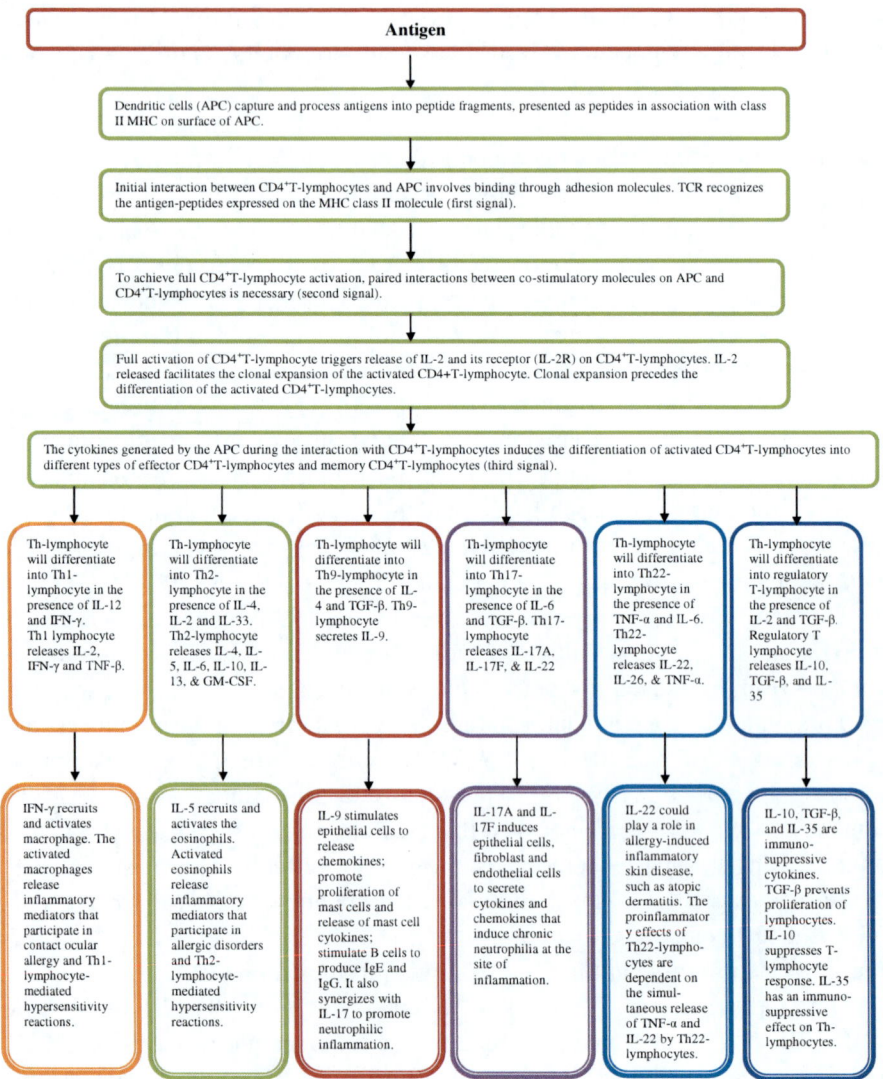

Figure 1a. T-Lymphocyte Activation.

In the presence of TNF-α and IL-6, CD4⁺T-lymphocytes express aryl hydrocarbon receptor (AHR) and differentiate into Th22-lymphocytes that secrete Th22-lymphocyte-derived cytokine (IL-22 and TNF-α). AHR is a key transcription factor that induces differentiation of CD4+T-lymphocytes into Th22-lymphocytes [22, 33-35]. Keratinocytes of the skin and epithelial cells express IL-22 receptors, and as such, Th22-lymphocytes could play a role in allergy-induced inflammatory skin disease, such as atopic dermatitis [32]. It should be noted that most of the proinflammatory effects of Th22-lymphocytes are dependent on the simultaneous release of TNF-α and IL-22 by Th22-lymphocytes [36].

The generation of induced regulatory T-lymphocytes occurs when IL-2 and TGF-β (produced by activated dendritic cells) in the presence of STAT5 induces the expression of Forkhead box P3 (FOXP3) on CD4⁺T-lymphocytes. FOXP3, an inducible regulatory T-lymphocyte transcription factor, induces the differentiation of CD4⁺T-lymphocytes into inducible regulatory T-lymphocytes that produce immunosuppressive cytokines, such as TGF-β, IL-10 and IL-35 [29, 37]. TGF-β prevents proliferation of lymphocytes whereas IL-10 suppresses T-lymphocyte response. IL-35 has an immuno-suppressive effect on Th-lymphocytes [13].

The development of the antibody-mediated immunity in allergic disorders usually involves the action of CD4⁺T-lymphocytes, B-lymphocytes, CD4⁺T-lymphocytes-derived cytokines, and antigen. In allergic disorders, antigen-specific activation of B-lymphocytes is CD4⁺T-lymphocyte dependent. To proliferate and differentiate into allergen-specific effector B-lymphocytes, two forms of signals are required. The first signal, provided by the B-cell coreceptor complex, occurs when an antigen binds to B-cell receptors (BCR). The antigen is internalized, processed, and presented as peptides in association with MHC class II molecules in the form of a antigen-peptide:MHC class II molecule complex on the surface of the B-lymphocyte. It is of note that the mature B-cell coreceptor complex is composed of four components: CD19, CD21 (complement receptor type 2, CR2), CD81 (target of antiproliferative antibody (TAPA)-1) and CD225 (LEU13, interferon-induced transmembrane protein 1) [12]. The other form of signal involves co-stimulation signals through CD40-CD40L interactions. Once the TCR recognizes the peptide-MHC class II molecule complex on the BCR, the CD4⁺T-lymphocyte will be stimulated to provide co-stimulation to the B-lymphocyte in the form of CD40L(CD154) on the CD4⁺T-lymphocyte engaging CD40 on the B-lymphocyte. CD40, a member of the TNF-receptor family of cytokine receptors, is involved in triggering B-lymphocyte proliferation and immunoglobulin class switching [12, 38].

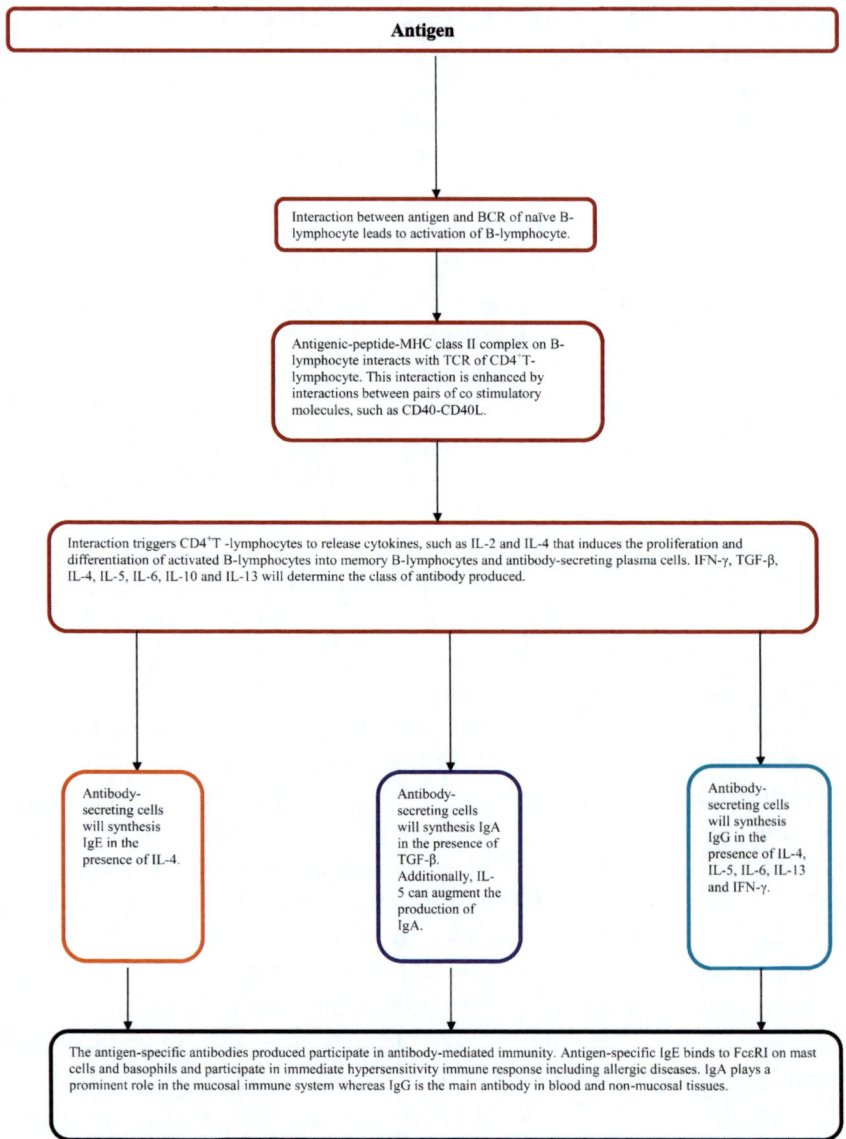

Figure 1b. B-Lymphocyte Activation.

The co-stimulatory CD40-CD40L interactions will induce the B-lymphocyte to upregulate the expression of B7 co-stimulatory molecules that ligate with CD28 receptors on the $CD4^+$T-lymphocyte. Additionally, it will lead to the upregulation of the surface receptor for B-cell stimulatory cytokines, such as IL-4, IL-5, IL-6, IFN-γ, and TGF-β that drives the proliferation and differentiation of B-lymphocyte into antibody-secreting plasma cells and memory B-lymphocytes. Antibody-secreting plasma cells are capable of secreting antibodies such as immunoglobulin G (IgG), IgA, IgM, IgE and IgD. IL-4 induces the production of IgG1 and IgE, while IFN-γ induces switching to IgG2a and IgG3. IL-5 augments the production of IgA, whereas TGF-β induces the production of IgA and IgG2b. The products of the proliferation and differentiation of the B-lymphocytes mediate the antibody-mediated immunity (figure 1b). IgE is involved in allergic disorders, whereas IgA is the major antibody in the mucosal immune system. IgG is the main antibody in blood and non-mucosal tissues [38, 39].

Immune Hypersensitivity Reaction in Allergic Eye Diseases

Antibody and cell-mediated immune hypersensitivity reaction occurs when the adaptive immune system overreacts in response to an antigen with consequential tissue damage [40]. A discussion of hypersensitivity reactions will be incomplete without briefly mentioning the Gell and Coomb's historic classification of hypersensitivity reactions. There are four types of immunological hypersensitivity reactions based on Gell and Coomb's classification. The first three types (types I-III) are antibody-mediated and type IV is mediated by T-lymphocytes. The IgE-mediated hypersensitivity (type I hypersensitivity) response is characterized by IgE-mediated mast cell degranulation with consequential release of inflammatory mediators [41, 42]. Type II hypersensitivity reaction is characterized by IgG antibodies binding to specific cell surface or matrix antigens. Type III hypersensitivity reaction occurs when IgG antibodies directed against widely distributed or soluble antigens lead to the formation of large quantities of soluble immune complexes or antigen-antibody aggregates [41, 43]. The T cell-mediated (type IV) hypersensitivity response is characterized by interactions of antigen with antigen specific T-lymphocytes with subsequent activation of T-lymphocytes to synthesize cytokines that recruit and activate inflammatory mediators [41].

The tissue damage that occurs in T-cell mediated hypersensitivity reactions occurs because of the recruitment and activation of eosinophils, macrophages and neutrophils. Mast cells and T-lymphocytes are considered the key cellular components of allergic disorders of the ocular surface.

The immune hypersensitivity mechanisms involved in allergic disorders include IgE-mediated hypersensitivity response, IgG-mediated hypersensitivity reactions and T-lymphocyte-mediated hypersensitivity response [42]. Antibody-mediated hypersensitivity reactions are characterized by allergen-induced mast cell activation and include IgG-and IgE-mediated hypersensitivity reactions. Antigen-mediated mast cell activation plays an important role in the initiation of cellular reaction in ocular allergy [44]. Human mast cells exposed to IFN-γ up-regulate the high affinity IgG receptor (FcγR) [45], whereas human mast cells exposed to Th2-derived cytokines such as IL-4 will express the high affinity IgE receptor (FcεRI) [46, 47]. The biologic consequence of recruiting mast cells into the site of inflammation through IgG-dependent activation is similar to those observed following IgE-dependent activation. Allergen-induced aggregation of receptor-bound IgE or IgG on the sensitized mast cell leads to mast cell degranulation, culminating in the release of granule-associated mediators, lipid mediators, chemokines and cytokines [45, 48, 49].

IgE-Mediated Hypersensitivity Reaction in Allergic Eye Diseases

The immune hypersensitivity mechanisms that will be discussed in this chapter are IgE-mediated hypersensitivity and T-lymphocyte mediated hypersensitivity. The mechanism of the IgE-mediated ocular allergic response occurs in three phases: the sensitization process, the early phase response, and the late phase response. The early-phase reaction lasts for 20-40 minutes following ocular allergen challenge, while the late phase response occurs approximately 4-6 hours after the early phase response [50]. The three phases of IgE-mediated hypersensitivity reactions include antigen-driven IgE production and the binding of antigen-specific IgE to the high affinity IgE receptors (FcεRI) on mast cells (sensitization phase); re-exposure of the ocular surface to allergen that induces mast cell degranulation with release of allergic mediators, a biochemical process mediated by allergen-driven cross-linking of IgE bound to FcεRI on sensitized mast cells (activation phase); and the clinical manifestations of the early and late phase response, attributable to the effects of the mediators released following mast cell activation (effector phase) [51]. The phases of the ocular allergic response are discussed below.

Sensitization Phase of Ocular Allergy

This occurs on initial exposure of the ocular surface to allergens. When deposited on the conjunctival mucosal epithelium, the environmental allergens are captured and processed by the APC into peptide fragments, which are then displayed on the surface of the APC in association with the major histocompatibility complex class II molecules [52, 53].

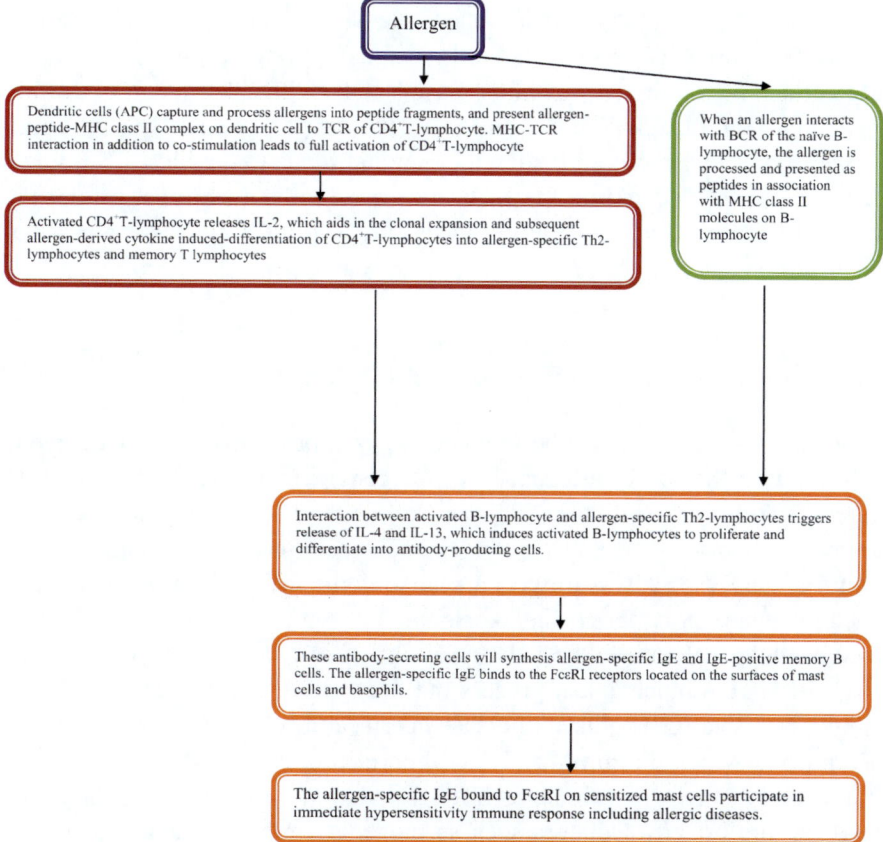

Figure 2. Sensitization Phase of Ocular Allergic Response.

The peptide fragment/MHC II complex on surface of the APC interacts with TCR on the naïve CD4$^+$ T-lymphocytes. The TCR-MHC interaction in conjunction with paired interactions between costimulatory molecules on the APC and naïve CD4$^+$T-lymphocytes leads to the activation of the naïve CD4$^+$ T-lymphocytes, and its subsequent differentiation into allergen-specific Th2-lymphocytes [52]. Additionally, the naïve B-lymphocyte interacts with the allergen and processes it into allergen peptides that is presented in association with MHC class II molecules in the form of allergen-peptide:MHC class II molecule complex on the BCR. The interaction between TCR of the allergen-specific Th2-lymphocytes and allergen-peptide:MHC class II molecule complex on B-lymphocytes in conjunction with co-stimulation signals through CD40-CD40L interactions triggers the release of Th2-lymphocyte derived cytokines (IL-4, IL-5, IL-6, IL-10, and IL-13). The B-lymphocytes, which recognized the same allergen that induced the Th2-lymphocyte differentiation, will in the presence of IL-4 and other signals from accessory molecules differentiate into antibody-producing plasma cells, with subsequent production of allergen-specific IgE [27, 41, 54, 55]. The allergen-specific IgE produced becomes specific for that particular allergen and binds to the high affinity IgE receptors (FcεRI) located on the surface of mast cells, a step that primes the mast cell for subsequent allergen exposure, completing the process of sensitization (figure 2) [8].

Early Phase Response (EPR) of Ocular Allergy

An allergic reaction will be initiated, when a previously sensitized eye is re-exposed to the same allergen. The allergens activate Th2-lymphocyte to express Th2-derived cytokines [56], as well as bind to the IgE molecules on the FcεRI receptors on the surface of the sensitized mast cells leading to cross linking of FcεRI [55]. This triggers a change in the mast cell outer membrane, which renders it more permeable to calcium ions with subsequent mobilization of intracellular calcium [52, 57, 58]. The influx of calcium ion into the mast cells initiates the biochemical process that leads to degranulation of the mast cell [59, 60]. The IgE-mediated increased permeability causes the mast cells to degranulate, which in turn, leads to the release of pro-allergic and pro-inflammatory mediators. Mast cell degranulation leads to the immediate release of preformed mediators such as biogenic amines (histamine), neutral proteases (chymase, tryptase), proteoglycans (heparin), and acid hydrolases, as well as the activation of phospholipase A2 to release arachidonic acid metabolites from membrane phospholipids within minutes of mast cell activation. Additionally, mast cell activation is associated with the release of cytokines (IL-4, IL-5, IL-6, IL-9, IL-13, TNF-α, TGF-β, and granulocyte macrophage-colony-stimulating factor (GM-CSF)), growth factors (bFGF, VEGF) and chemokines (CXCL8, CCL2 (MCP-1), CCL3, CCL5 (RANTES), and CCL11 (eotaxin)). The mast cell-derived cytokines activates vascular endothelial cells to express chemokines and adhesion molecules [47, 61].

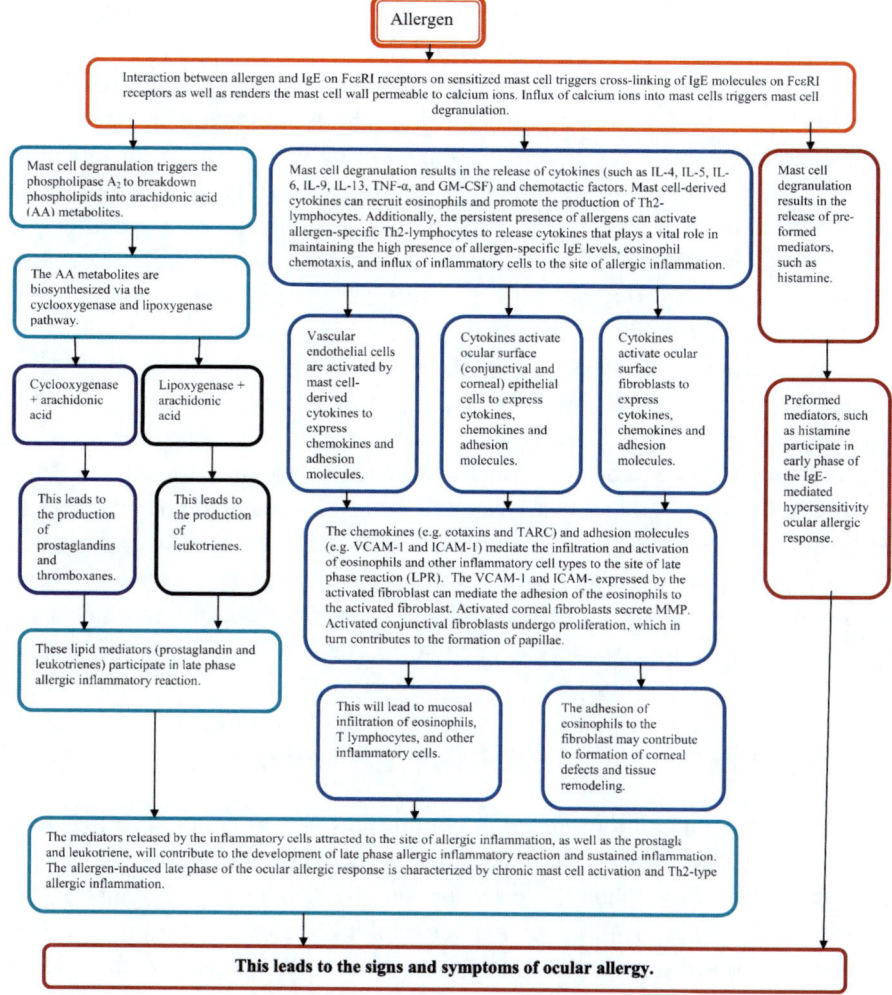

Figure 3. The Early and Late Phase Response of Ocular Allergic Response.

The preformed mediators are primarily responsible for the early phase symptoms, which last for approximately 40 minutes following initial exposure. The histamine released stimulates the blood vessels (H1 and H2 receptors on vascular smooth muscles), nerves (H1 receptors on nerve endings), and mucous-producing glands (H1 receptors on glandular cells) resulting in the hallmark signs and symptoms of ocular allergy (redness, itching, tearing, chemosis and eyelid edema) [27, 62]. The AA metabolites are then biosynthesized through the cyclooxygenase pathway into prostaglandins (PGD2, PGE1, PGE2) and thromboxanes, and via the lipoxygenase pathway into leukotrienes (LTB4, LTC4, LTD4, LTE4) [63]. Thymus- and activation-regulated chemokine (TARC), a potent chemoattractant for Th2-lymphocytes, mediate the recruitment of allergen-specific Th2-lymphocytes to the site of allergic inflammation. Additionally, the continuous presence of allergen activates allergen-specific Th2-lymphocytes to produce IL-4, IL-5, IL-9, and IL-13, which plays a role in the maintenance of high allergen-specific IgE levels. These cytokines also recruit and activate eosinophil, as well as induces influx of inflammatory cells into the site of allergic inflammation [19]. Cytokines activate ocular surface (conjunctival and corneal) epithelial cells and fibroblasts to express chemokines and adhesion molecules. The chemokines (e.g. eotaxins and TARC) and adhesion molecules (e.g. VCAM-1 and ICAM-1) mediate the recruitment of eosinophils and other inflammatory cell types into the site of allergic inflammation [47, 61]. Additionally, VCAM-1 and ICAM- expressed by the activated fibroblast can mediate the adhesion of the eosinophils to the activated fibroblast [64]. Thus, the mast cell-derived cytokines and chemokines as well as the lipid mediators contribute to the development of the late phase allergic inflammatory reaction and sustained inflammation at the site of allergic reaction (figure 3) [41].

Late Phase Response (LPR) of Ocular Allergy

The LPR of the allergic reaction commences 4 to 6 hours after the mast cell releases its pre-formed and newly formed mediators [65]. This response is characterized by T-lymphocyte activation and the release of Th2-lymphocyte-derived cytokines. It is of note that chemokines released during the EPR mediate the recruitment and activation of inflammatory cells to the site of allergic reaction, resulting in the infiltration of the conjunctiva with eosinophils, neutrophils, T-lymphocytes, and monocytes [27, 54, 62, 66-68]. The eosinophils release their enzymes and toxic granule products (e.g.

EMBP), which are capable of inducing a chronic allergic inflammatory response typical of a Th2-mediated DTH/LPR [62, 68-71]. The mediators released by nonimmune cells and inflammatory cells attracted to the site of allergic inflammation, as well as the prostaglandin and leukotriene, will contribute to the chronic allergic inflammatory reaction seen in LPR (figure 3). LPR is a persistent process that intensifies the allergic inflammation and heightens the entire allergic mechanism, thus prolonging the allergic expression [27, 41]. The release of histamine by mast cell in LPR by chemokines and cytokines produced by inflammatory cells such as eosinophils and neutrophils [52, 72], and the activation of vascular endothelial cells, epithelial cells and fibroblasts are other mechanisms that may intensify the allergic inflammation [27, 62]. The LPR is an essential aspect of the immunopathology of chronic ocular allergy. The LPR effects are the major cause of ocular surface damage, such as keratitis, limbal infiltration, tissue remodeling, and corneal ulcer that occurs in the ocular allergy [53].

T-Lymphocyte-Mediated Hypersensitivity in Allergic Eye Diseases

T-lymphocyte mediated hypersensitivity response occurs when allergen react with antigen-specific sensitized T-lymphocytes with consequential release of cytokines and chemokines. It occurs in two phases - sensitization and elicitation phase. The sensitization phase occurs when APC present processed allergen-peptide:MHC class II complex to T-lymphocytes with consequential differentiation of CD4$^+$T- lymphocytes into effector CD4$^+$ T-lymphocytes and memory Th-lymphocytes. Effector CD8$^+$T-lymphocytes are generated when allergen-peptide:MHC class I complex interacts with T-lymphocytes. The focus in this chapter will be on Th-lymphocyte-mediated hypersensitivity reactions. Re-exposure following earlier priming will trigger the elicitation phase of type IV hypersensitivity reaction. During the elicitation phase, activation and proliferation of memory Th-lymphocytes occurs when the TCR on the memory Th-lymphocytes recognizes the allergen peptide-MHC class II complex on APC. The activated Th-lymphocytes release cytokines and chemokines that mediate Th-lymphocyte mediated hypersensitivity response [69, 73]. The activated Th1-lymphocytes release chemokines and cytokines that mediate the clinicopathological features of Th1-lymphocyte mediated hypersensitivity reaction. Th1-lymphocyte-derived cytokines and chemokines induces the recruitment of monocytes to the site of inflammation, where they undergo maturation into tissue macrophages that are capable of acting as antigen presenting cells to the memory Th1-lymphocytes [69]. TNF-α and TNF-β released by the activated Th1-lymphocytes can cause local tissue destruction and up-regulate the expression of adhesion molecules on local blood vessels. IL-3 and GM-CSF stimulates the production of tissue macrophages from monocytes. The IFN-γ released by the activated Th1-lymphocyte will induce the expression of vascular adhesion molecules as well as activate macrophages to release proteases, TNF-α, reactive oxygen intermediates, and nitric oxide that cause Th1-mediated tissue damage [13, 69]. Additionally, the activated macrophage may fuse to form multinucleated giant cells and/or make epithelioid cells that play a role in the formation of chronic granuloma. The activated Th2-lymphocyte releases IL-4 and IL-5 that play a major role in Th2-lymphocyte mediated DTH. IL-5 stimulates the chemotaxis and activation of eosinophil to the site of inflammation [69]. The activated eosinophil degranulates to secrete enzymes, lipid mediators and toxic granule proteins that can cause significant tissue damage in ocular allergy [13, 69]. IL-4 plays a significant role in Th2-lymphocyte mediated DTH characterized by chronic IgE production and mast cell activation. Thus, Th2-lymphocyte mediated DTH plays a role in atopic dermatitis and late phase response of ocular allergy [70].

Th9-lymphocyte-derived cytokine, IL-9 is capable of activating mast cells to release proinflammatory cytokines [21]. It also induces epithelial cells to release chemokines that facilitate eosinophil and T-lymphocyte infiltration. These effector actions of Th9-lymphocytes could perpetuate the chronic allergic inflammation as well as cause Th9-lymphocyte-mediated hypersensitivity reaction [29, 30].

Recent studies have suggested that IL-17 and IL-22 secreted by Th17-lymphocyte and Th22-lymphocyte respectively play a role in sustained inflammation in allergic diseases [32]. Th17-lymphocyte secretes IL-17, a cytokine that is capable of stimulating epithelial cells and fibroblast to express cytokines, adhesion molecules and chemokines. It stimulates epithelial cells to express IL-6, IL-8, CXCL1, CXCL6, ICAM-1, and MUC5AC, whereas stimulated fibroblast will express IL-6, IL-8, CXCL1, and ICAM-1. Additionally, it activates macrophages to release IL-1β, TNF-α, and MMP-9, which are known to cause inflammation and tissue damage. Furthermore, IL-17 induces keratinocytes to release IL-6 and IL-8. Thus, Th17-lymphocyte through its effector function could facilitate the infiltration of eosinophils, macrophages and neutrophils into the site of allergic inflammation, leading to

Th17-lymphocyte mediated hypersensitivity reaction, as well as Th17-lymphocyte mediated tissue inflammation in patients with allergic contact dermatitis [74]. Because Th22-lymphocytes co-express CCR6 and the skin-homing receptors CCR4 and CCR10, they can participate in Th22-lymphocyte mediated tissue inflammation in chronic atopic dermatitis [32]. The proinflammatory effects of Th22-lymphocytes are mostly dependent on the simultaneous release of TNF-α and IL-22 by Th22-lymphocyte [34, 36].

References

[1]   Delves, P., et al., Innate Immunity, in Roitt's Essential Immunology. 2011, *Wiley-Blackwell.* p. 3-34.

[2]   Beutler, B., Innate immunity: an overview. *Mol Immunol,* 2004. 40(12): p. 845-59.

[3]   Li, D., et al., Recent Advances in Mucosal Immunology and Ocular Surface Diseases, in Advances in Ophthalmology, S. Rumelt, Editor 2012. p. 49-78.

[4]   Heine, H., TLRs, NLRs and RLRs: innate sensors and their impact on allergic diseases--a current view. *Immunol Lett,* 2011. 139(1-2): p. 14-24.

[5]   Staros, E.B., Innate immunity: New approaches to understanding its clinical significance. *Am J Clin Pathol,* 2005. 123(2): p. 305-12.

[6]   Chang, J.H., P.J. McCluskey, and D. Wakefield, Toll-like receptors in ocular immunity and the immunopathogenesis of inflammatory eye disease. *Br J Ophthalmol,* 2006. 90(1): p. 103-8.

[7]   Murphy, K.P., Travers, P., Walport, M., Innate Immunity: The First Lines of Defense, in Janeway's Immunobiology. 2012, Garland Science: New York. p. 37-74.

[8]   Goodman, J.W., The Immune Response. In: Stites DP, Terr AI, editors. Basic Human Immunology., ed. T.A. Stites DP. 1991.: *Appleton and Lange.* 34-44.

[9]   Siminovitch, K., The new immunology. *J Reconstr Microsurg,* 1992. 8(2): p. 121-9.

[10]   Male, D.R., Ivan. , Adaptive and Innate Immunity. In: Roitt I, Brostoff J, Male D, editors. Immunology., ed. B.J. Roitt I, Male D. 1989 St. Louis: *The C.V. Mosby* Co. 1.1-1.10. .

[11]   Lanier, L., Cells of the Immune Response: Lymphocytes and Mononuclear Phagocytes. In: Stites DP, Terr AI, editors. Basic Human

Immunology. , ed. T.A. Stites DP. 1991, Norwalk, Connecticut: *Appleton and Lange.* 61-72

[12] Delves, P., et al., Lymphocyte Activation, in Roitt's Essential Immunology. 2011, *Wiley-Blackwell.* p. 205-225.

[13] Murphy, K.P., Travers, P., Walport, M., T Cell-Mediated Immunity, in Janeway's Immunobiology. 2012, *Garland Science:* New York. p. 335-386.

[14] Murphy, K.P., Travers, P., Walport, M., Antigen Recognition by B-cell and T-cell Receptors, in Janeway's Immunobiology. 2012, *Garland Science:* New York. p. 127-156.

[15] Takesono, A., L.D. Finkelstein, and P.L. Schwartzberg, Beyond calcium: new signaling pathways for Tec family kinases. *J Cell Sci,* 2002. 115(Pt 15): p. 3039-48.

[16] Readinger, J.A., et al., Tec kinases regulate T-lymphocyte development and function: new insights into the roles of Itk and Rlk/Txk. *Immunol Rev,* 2009. 228(1): p. 93-114.

[17] Murphy, K.P., Travers, P., Walport, M., Signalimg Through Immune-System Receptors, in Janeway's Immunobiology. 2012, *Garland Science:* New York. p. 239-274.

[18] Almawi, W.Y. and O.K. Melemedjian, Molecular mechanisms of glucocorticoid antiproliferative effects: antagonism of transcription factor activity by glucocorticoid receptor. *J Leukoc Biol,* 2002. 71(1): p. 9-15.

[19] Akkoc, T., M. Akdis, and C.A. Akdis, Update in the mechanisms of allergen-specific immunotheraphy. *Allergy Asthma Immunol Res,* 2011. 3(1): p. 11-20.

[20] Vock, C., H.P. Hauber, and M. Wegmann, The other T helper cells in asthma pathogenesis. *J Allergy* (Cairo), 2010. 2010: p. 519298.

[21] Jager, A. and V.K. Kuchroo, Effector and regulatory T-cell subsets in autoimmunity and tissue inflammation. *Scand J Immunol,* 2010. 72(3): p. 173-84.

[22] Annunziato, F. and S. Romagnani, Heterogeneity of human effector CD4+ T cells. *Arthritis Res Ther,* 2009. 11(6): p. 257.

[23] Delves, P.J.M., Seamus J.; Burton, Dennis R.; Roitt, Ivan M. , The Production of Effectors. Roitt's Essential Immunology. 2006: *Blackwell Publishing.* 185-210.

[24] Marini, J.C., Cell Cooperation in Antibody Response. In: Male D, Brostoff J, Roth DB, Roitt I, editors. Immunology., ed. B.J. Male D, Roth DB, Roitt I. 2006: *Mosby Elsevier.* 163-180.

[25] Bonini, S., A. Lambiase, and M. Sacchetti, Cytokines in ocular allergy. *Int Ophthalmol Clin, 2003*. 43(1): p. 27-32.

[26] Uchio, E., et al., Tear levels of interferon-gamma, interleukin (IL) -2, IL-4 and IL-5 in patients with vernal keratoconjunctivitis, atopic keratoconjunctivitis and allergic conjunctivitis. *Clin Exp Allergy, 2000*. 30(1): p. 103-9.

[27] Leonardi, A., Pathophysiology of allergic conjunctivitis. *Acta Ophthalmol Scand Suppl*, 1999(228): p. 21-3.

[28] Tan, C. and I. Gery, The unique features of Th9 cells and their products. *Crit Rev Immunol, 2012*. 32(1): p. 1-10.

[29] Stassen, M., E. Schmitt, and T. Bopp, From interleukin-9 to T helper 9 cells. *Ann N Y Acad Sci, 2012*. 1247: p. 56-68.

[30] Soroosh, P. and T.A. Doherty, Th9 and allergic disease. *Immunology,* 2009. 127(4): p. 450-8.

[31] Jutel, M. and C.A. Akdis, T-cell subset regulation in atopy. *Curr Allergy Asthma Rep*, 2011. 11(2): p. 139-45.

[32] Souwer, Y., et al., IL-17 and IL-22 in atopic allergic disease. *Curr Opin Immunol, 2010*. 22(6): p. 821-6.

[33] Zhang, N., H.F. Pan, and D.Q. Ye, Th22 in inflammatory and autoimmune disease: prospects for therapeutic intervention. *Mol Cell Biochem, 2011*. 353(1-2): p. 41-6.

[34] Eyerich, S., et al., Th22 cells represent a distinct human T cell subset involved in epidermal immunity and remodeling. *J Clin Invest, 2009*. 119(12): p. 3573-85.

[35] Ramirez, J.M., et al., Activation of the aryl hydrocarbon receptor reveals distinct requirements for IL-22 and IL-17 production by human T helper cells. *Eur J Immunol, 2010*. 40(9): p. 2450-9.

[36] Cavani, A., D. Pennino, and K. Eyerich, Th17 and Th22 in skin allergy. *Chem Immunol Allergy, 2012*. 96: p. 39-44.

[37] Wong, M.T., et al., Regulation of human Th9 differentiation by type I interferons and IL-21. *Immunol Cell Biol, 2010*. 88(6): p. 624-31.

[38] Murphy, K.P., Travers, P., Walport, M., The Humoral Immune Response, in Janeway's Immunobiology. 2012, *Garland Science:* New York. p. 387-428.

[39] Delves, P., et al., The Production of Effectors in Roitt's Essential Immunology. 2011, *Wiley-Blackwell.* p. 226-262.

[40] Schmid, K.L. and L.M. Schmid, Ocular allergy: causes and therapeutic options. *Clin Exp Optom, 2000*. 83(5): p. 257-270.

[41] Chigbu, D.I., The pathophysiology of ocular allergy: a review. *Cont Lens Anterior Eye,* 2009. 32(1): p. 3-15; quiz 43-4.

[42] Terr, A.I., Mechanism of Hypersensitivity In: Stites DP, Terr AI, Parslow TG, editors. Basic and Clinical Immunology., ed. T.A. Stites DP, Parslow TG. 1994, Norwalk, Connecticut:: *Appleton and Lange.* 314-326.

[43] Murphy, K.P., Travers, P., Walport, M., Allergy and Allergic Diseases, in Janeway's Immunobiology. 2012, *Garland Science:* New York. p. 571-610.

[44] Tkaczyk, C., et al., Fcgamma receptors on mast cells: activatory and inhibitory regulation of mediator release. *Int Arch Allergy Immunol,* 2004. 133(3): p. 305-15.

[45] Woolhiser, M., K. Brockow, and D. Metcalfe, Activation of human mast cells by aggregated IgG through FcgammaRI: additive effects of C3a. *Clin Immunol,* 2004. 110(2): p. 172-80.

[46] Toru, H., et al., Induction of the high-affinity IgE receptor (Fc epsilon RI) on human mast cells by IL-4. *Int Immunol,* 1996. 8(9): p. 1367-73.

[47] Brown, J., T. Wilson, and D. Metcalfe, The mast cell and allergic diseases: role in pathogenesis and implications for therapy. *Clin Exp Allergy,* 2008. 38(1): p. 4-18.

[48] Tkaczyk, C., et al., Activation of human mast cells through the high affinity IgG receptor. *Mol Immunol,* 2002. 38(16-18): p. 1289-93.

[49] Woolhiser, M., et al., IgG-dependent activation of human mast cells following up-regulation of FcgammaRI by IFN-gamma. *Eur J Immunol,* 2001. 31(11): p. 3298-307.

[50] Solomon, A., J. Pe'er, and F. Levi-Schaffer, Advances in ocular allergy: basic mechanisms, clinical patterns and new therapies. *Curr Opin Allergy Clin Immunol,* 2001. 1(5): p. 477-82.

[51] Benjamin, E., R. Coico, and G. Sunshine, Hypersensitivity reactions: Antibody-Mediated (Type I) reactions. *Immunology A Short Course.* 2000, New York: Wiley-Liss. 279-300.

[52] Ohbayashi, M., et al., The Role of Histamine in Ocular Allergy. *Adv Exp Med Biol,* 2010. 709: p. 43-52.

[53] Abelson, M.B.L., A.; Smith, L., The Mechanisms, Diagnosis and Treatment of Allergy. *Review of Ophthalmology,* 2002. 9 (4): p. 74- 84.

[54] Hendricks, R.L. and Q. Tang, Cellular Immunity and the Eye In: Pepose JS, Holland GN, Wilhelmus KR, editors. *Ocular Infection and Immunity.* 1996, St Louis: Mosby. 71-95.

[55]   Butrus, S. and R. Portela, Ocular allergy: diagnosis and treatment. *Ophthalmol Clin North Am,* 2005. 18(4): p. 485-92, v.

[56]   Broide, D.H., Immunomodulation of allergic disease. *Annu Rev Med,* 2009. 60: p. 279-91.

[57]   Berdy, G., Atopic keratoconjunctivitis (AKC). *Acta Ophthalmol Scand Suppl,* 1999(228): p. 7-9.

[58]   Tabbara, K., Immunopathogenesis of chronic allergic conjunctivitis. *Int Ophthalmol Clin,* 2003. 43(1): p. 1-7.

[59]   Terr, A.I., Mechanism of Inflammation. In: Stites DP, Terr AI, editors. Basic Human Immunology. 1991, Norwalk, Connecticut: *Appleton and Lange.* 131-140.

[60]   Reiss, J., et al., Allergic conjunctivitis. In: Pepose JS, Holland GN, Wilhelmus KR, editors. *Ocular infection and immunity.* 1996, St. Louis: Mosby. 345–58.

[61]   Irani, A.M., Ocular mast cells and mediators. *Immunol Allergy Clin North Am,* 2008. 28(1): p. 25-42, v.

[62]   Abelson, M.B., L. Smith, and M. Chapin, Ocular allergic disease: mechanisms, disease sub-types, treatment. *Ocul Surf,* 2003. 1(3): p. 127-49.

[63]   Howarth, P., Antihistamines in rhinoconjunctivitis. *Clin Allergy Immunol,* 2002. 17: p. 179-220.

[64]   Okada, N., et al., The implications of the upregulation of ICAM-1/VCAM-1 expression of corneal fibroblasts on the pathogenesis of allergic keratopathy. *Invest Ophthalmol Vis Sci,* 2005. 46(12): p. 4512-8.

[65]   Epstein, A.B., New Horizons in Ocular Allergy. *Review of Optometry,* 2002. 139(3): p. 117-124.

[66]   Leonardi, A., Emerging drugs for ocular allergy. *Expert Opin Emerg Drugs,* 2005. 10(3): p. 505-20.

[67]   Durham, S., The inflammatory nature of allergic disease. *Clin Exp Allergy,* 1998. 28 Suppl 6: p. 20-4.

[68]   Askenase, P., Proposing Th2 DTH relevant to asthma: cutaneous basophil hypersensitivity then and now. *Chem Immunol,* 2000. 78: p. 112-23.

[69]   Delves, P., et al., Allergy and Other hypersensitivities, in Roitt's Essential Immunology. 2011, *Wiley-Blackwell.* p. 394-422.

[70]   Romagnani, S., Lymphokine production by human T cells in disease states. *Annu Rev Immunol,* 1994. 12: p. 227-57.

[71] Cousins, S.W. and B.T. Rouse, Chemical Mediators of Ocular Inflammation In: Pepose JS, Holland GN, Wilhelmus KR, editors. *Ocular Infection and Immunity.* 1996, St Louis: Mosby. 50-70.

[72] Bielory, L. and S. Ghafoor, Histamine receptors and the conjunctiva. *Curr Opin Allergy Clin Immunol,* 2005. 5(5): p. 437-40.

[73] Nelson, J., C. Mowad, and H. Sun, Allergic Contact Dermatitis and Patch-Testing Education in US Dermatology Residencies in 2010. *Dermatitis,* 2012. 23(2): p. 56-60.

[74] Oboki, K., et al., Th17 and allergy. *Allergol Int,* 2008. 57(2): p. 121-34.

Chapter 5

Pharmacotherapy of Allergic Ocular Surface Diseases

The management options of allergic disorders of the ocular surface ranges from non-pharmacologic strategies to the use of pharmaceutical agents. The primary treatment for allergic eye conditions in general is removal of the offending agent, which in turn, prevents the onset of allergic eye response. However, when non-pharmacologic approach fails to control the ocular allergic expression, the clinician should initiate pharmacological management modalities [1]. This chapter would review most of the pharmaceutical agents used in the management of allergic disorders of the ocular surface.

Vasoconstrictors

Antihistamine/vasoconstrictor combinations contain both an antihistamine (e.g. antazoline phosphate) and vasoconstrictor (e.g. naphazoline or phenylepherine). The antihistamines in these topical agents help to decrease the itch associated with allergic conjunctivitis. The vasoconstrictors in these agents are adrenergic agonists that stimulate α-adrenoreceptors. They are capable of reducing the chemosis, redness and eyelid edema resulting from tissue congestion [2]. Antihistamine/vasoconstrictor combination agents are indicated for relieving the symptoms and signs of allergic conjunctivitis. They are relatively fast acting but the duration of action lasts only 2 to 4 hours. Dosing more frequently has the potential to cause adverse effects [2-4]. Because these agents have a limited duration of action, and as such, they may not provide all day therapeutic effect [5]. The adverse effects of these agents include burning and stinging on instillation; mydriasis, especially in patients with lighter irides; follicular conjunctivitis; eczematoid blepharoconjunctivitis and rebound hyperemia or conjunctivitis medicamentosa (an allergic reaction to the agent itself) with long-term use [2]. The clinician should use caution when prescribing vasoconstrictors to patients with cardiovascular disease, hyperthyroidism or angle-closure glaucoma. In the management of ocular allergy, this should not be of major concern, as they are more suitable and superior alternatives to antihistamine/vasoconstrictor agents. The non-specificity of the pharmacologic action of antihistamine/vasoconstrictors combination agents in dealing with the ocular allergic response and its adverse ocular effects makes it inappropriate for long-term use [3, 6].

Antihistamines

In general, first-generation oral H1 receptor antagonists, such as chlorphenamine or cyclizine possess both symptom relieving and sedating effects. However, second-generation agents are non-sedating. The sedative effect is due to their lipophilic nature, which allows first-generation agents to cross the blood–brain barrier and inhibit the central neurotransmitter effects of histamine. The first-generation H1 antagonists have reduced specificity for H1 receptors, and as such, this results in a degree of peripheral muscarinic and α-adrenergic blockade. The most serious adverse side effect of the first generation antihistamines is cardiotoxicity in the form of an increase in the QT interval and a tendency towards cardiac arrhythmia. The second-generation drugs (such as cetirizine, desloratidine, fexofenadine and loratidine) have safer cardiac side effect profiles [1]. H1-antihistamines are widely used in the treatment of various allergic diseases. Cetirizine is a piperazine derivative, whereas fexofenadine and loratadine are piperidine derivatives [7]. Cetirizine hydrochloride, a piperazine derivative and carboxylated metabolite of hydroxyzine, is a potent selective H1 receptor antagonist with the added feature of inhibiting histamine release and eosinophil chemotaxis. It is an effective and well-tolerated antihistamine for patients with allergic rhinoconjunctivitis. The low sedative potential of cetirizine makes it a useful alternative to oral antihistamines with high sedative potential [8, 9]. Loratadine is a long acting, potent antihistamine that is chemically related to the tricyclic antidepressants with a threefold greater affinity for peripheral than central H1-receptors. It exhibits low sedative potential, as well as low incidence of anticholinergic side effects [10]. Descarbethoxyloratadine, the main metabolite of Loratadine, is four times more active than the parent drug [11]. The anti-allergic properties of loratadine could be attributed to its direct inhibitory effect on eosinophil activation [12]. Loratadine is a well-tolerated and fast acting antihistamine that is safe and efficacious in treating patients with seasonal allergic rhinitis [10, 13].

Topical H1 antagonists have much lower systemic absorption, and as such, they have fewer side effects than their oral counterparts. The second-generation topical H1 receptor antagonists have a prolonged clinical effect. Oral antihistamines have a slower onset of action than topical agents and may cause ocular and systemic adverse effects. Topical treatment is, therefore, preferable for isolated allergic eye disease [1].

The new generation topical antihistamines such as levocabastine 0.05% and emedastine 0.05% are superior to the first generation topical antihistamines (pheniramine and antazoline) and work by competitively blocking histamine receptors on the ocular mucosal surface [2]. The first generation topical antihistamines have limited potency whereas the newer antihistamines have longer duration and are well tolerated [3]. Levocabastine HCl ophthalmic suspension 0.05 %, a cyclohexy-3-methylpiperidine derivative, is a potent topical selective H1-receptor antihistamine suspension with rapid onset of action of 15 minutes and prolonged clinical effect lasting up to 4 hours [14]. It has been shown, in an ocular allergen challenge model, to downregulate intracellular adhesion molecules by almost 50%. It has a recommended dosage regimen of one drop to be administered four-times-daily [1]. The main adverse events seen are ocular irritation, dry eyes and dry mouth after application of eye drops [14]. Emedastine difumarate 0.05% ophthalmic solution is a safe and potent selective histamine H1-receptor antagonist with no apparent effects on adrenergic, dopaminergic or serotonin receptors [15]. The enhanced potency of emedastine difumarate is attributed to its ability to inhibit cytokine secretion by the epithelial cells [16]. It is indicated for the temporary relief of the signs and symptoms associated with allergic conjunctivitis [17]. It is also recommended at a dosage of four-times-daily and the side effect may include mild burning or stinging sensation. Clinical studies comparing ketotifen and emedastine suggested that emedastine and ketotifen are not significantly different with respect to anti-itching efficacy in the CAC model of acute allergic conjunctivitis [18, 19].

Mast Cell Stabilizers

Topical mast cell stabilizers prevent the release of allergic mediators from mast cells by suppressing mast cell degranulation. The blockade of mast cell degranulation inhibits the release of preformed and newly formed mediators of allergy [2, 20]. They also achieve their clinical effect by preventing calcium influx across the cell membrane [21, 22]. Mast cell stabilizers are safe and effective for the long-term therapeutic management of allergic eye diseases. They require a loading time of up to two weeks since it has no effect on acute allergic reactions induced by histamine already released on the ocular surface [6, 23].

Sodium cromoglycate is a mast cell stabilizer that is suitable for long-term prophylaxis and therapeutic management of ocular allergy. It is not effective in inhibiting the degranulation of mucosal mast cells. This may explain the poor response of chronic ocular allergies to sodium cromoglycate [22]. The efficacy of the medication seems to be dependent on the concentration of the solution used [1]. The major adverse effect is burning and stinging. The 4% formulation is dosed four to six times daily, and tapered to twice daily when symptoms subside [2].

Lodoxamide tromethamine 0.1% ophthalmic solution possesses mast cell stabilizing properties that are considered to be 2500 times more potent than that of sodium cromolyn [2]. The anti-allergic properties of lodoxamide are attributed to its ability to inhibit eosinophil activation and production of leukotrienes [24, 25]. It is safe for use in children and adults on a four-times-daily dosing for up to 3 months. The most common side effects are burning and stinging [2]

Pemirolast potassium 0.1% ophthalmic solution, a pyridopyrimidine compound, is a mast cell stabilizer that is used for the treatment of seasonal allergic and vernal conjunctivitis. It is dosed four-times-daily and it is safe for use in children as young as 2 years of age [2]. Nedocromil sodium 2% ophthalmic solution, a pyranoquinoline dicarboxylic acid, is a potent stabilizer of both connective and mucosal type mast cells [2, 3]. It has been reported that mast cell stabilization by nedocromil sodium may be due to its ability to inhibit chloride ion flux in mast cells and epithelial cells [1]. Additionally, nedocromil sodium has H1 receptor antagonist properties and inhibitory effect on eosinophils, and as such, it could be considered a multi-action antiallergic agent [26]. Furthermore, it can reduce the expression of ICAM-1 by conjunctival epithelial cells [24, 26]. The inhibition of IgE production by B-lymphocytes may be an alternative pharmacological mechanism of nedocromil sodium [1, 27]. The tear levels of histamine and prostaglandins D2 are reduced following the administration of nedocromil sodium [24, 26]. In patients with chronic ocular allergies, twice-a-day dosed nedocromil sodium has been shown to be very effective at preventing release of allergic mediators from the mucosal type mast cell. Nedocromil sodium ophthalmic solution is an effective and well-tolerated anti-allergic agent for the long-term management of ocular allergies [28, 29]. It is associated with ocular stinging upon instillation and a distinctive taste [2].

Multimodal or Dual Acting Agents

Antihistamine/Mast cell Stabilizing combinations are multimodal anti-allergic agents that act as both histamine receptor antagonist and mast cell stabilizer. Olopatadine ophthalmic solution, epinastine ophthalmic solution, ketotifen ophthalmic solution, bepotastine besilate ophthalmic solution, alcaftadine ophthalmic solution, and azelastine ophthalmic solution are topical multimodal anti-allergic pharmaceutical agents. These agents reduce the allergic cascade by providing immediate symptomatic relief by blocking histamine receptors and inhibiting release of allergic mediators via stabilization of mast cells. The efficacy of multimodal agents with both antihistamine and mast cell stabilizing properties have been demonstrated with the conjunctival allergen challenge (CAC) model [30].

Olopatadine HCL (0.1% and 0.2%) ophthalmic solution is a multimodal anti-allergic agent that possesses selective H1-receptor antagonism and mast cell stabilizing features [2]. It has a rapid onset of action and prolonged clinical effect [31]. Olopatadine has potent H1-antagonist activity, and as such, it could attenuate histamine-stimulated phosphatidylinositol turnover and cytokine secretion by conjunctival epithelial cells [16]. Olopatadine stabilizes the mast cell, and as such, it prevents the release of pro-allergic and pro-inflammatory mediators [21, 32]. Olopatadine also inhibits IgE-mediated TNF-α release from conjunctival mast cells (MC_{TC} phenotype) and inhibits upregulation of ICAM-1 expression on epithelial cells, which in turn, results in a decrease in the recruitment of inflammatory cells [26]. Thus, the prolonged clinical effect of olopatadine could be attributed to its ability to suppress the release of pro-allergic and pro-inflammatory mediators. It reduces all signs and symptoms of allergic conjunctivitis, including redness, itching, chemosis, tearing and eyelid edema. Olopatadine is approved for the treatment of the signs and symptoms of allergic conjunctivitis [31, 33]. The olopatadine 0.1%

formulation is dosed twice daily whereas the olopatadine 0.2% formulation is dosed once daily. Multiple clinical studies have shown that olopatadine has exceptional duration of action, efficacy, and tolerability [30]. Olopatadine demonstrates clear efficacy for relieving ocular pruritus and has the advantage of having a more neutral PH with lower surface activity [34]. Furthermore, it has been demonstrated that olopatadine does not interfere with allergy skin testing making discontinuation in preparation for skin prick testing unnecessary [30]. It is of note that olopatadine can decrease the mucus discharge in VKC by reducing the goblet cell density in the conjunctiva. Several studies have shown that olopatadine 0.2% is effective for up to 24 hours after instillation when dosed once daily with a well-tolerated safety profile in adults and children of 3 years of age and older [15, 35].

Azelastine hydrochloride 0.05% ophthalmic solution, a phthalazinone derivative, is a twice-a-day dosed multiple-action anti-allergic agent [26]. It has a rapid onset of action and prolonged therapeutic effect. Azelastine is a potent H1 receptor antagonist that inhibits the early allergic response and mediator release by stabilizing the mast cell [24]. It downregulates ICAM-1 expression in the conjunctiva, and as such, it attenuates the ability of ICAM-1 to facilitate accumulation of inflammatory cells at the site of allergic reaction [36]. It attenuates the release of pro-inflammatory cytokines from conjunctival epithelial cells and mast cells [16]. Azelastine inhibits leukotriene production as well as the production of superoxide by neutrophils and eosinophils [26]. The preventive effect of azelastine is attributed to its ability to inhibit calcium ion mobilization and reduce accumulation of inflammatory cells at the site of allergic reaction during EPR and LPR [37]. Its anti-inflammatory properties appear to stem from its ability to inhibit mast cell mediator release, as well as inhibit leukotriene production [34]. Azelastine ophthalmic solution is indicated for the treatment of ocular itching associated with allergic conjunctivitis. It has a noticeable bitter taste and can cause ocular stinging upon instillation [2, 37, 38]. The unpleasant or bitter taste results from the passage of the drug down the lacrimal duct through the nasal cavity to the tongue [39]. It is approved for use in adults and children 3 years and older.

Ketotifen fumarate 0.025% ophthalmic solution, a benzocyclo-heptathiophene derivative, is a twice-a-day dosed multimodal anti-allergic agent with strong H1 receptor antagonist, mast cell stabilizing, and anti-mediator properties [2, 26, 40]. It has been demonstrated that ketotifen can reduce antigen-induced mast cell degranulation, and as such, it prevents the release of pro-allergic and pro-inflammatory mediators. Additionally, it prevents eosinophil accumulation [1, 15, 24, 26]. Ketotifen has been shown to have a biphasic effect on mast cell stabilization, in which it inhibits release of histamine from the mast cell at low or optimal effective inhibitory concentrations and stimulates histamine release at slightly higher than effective inhibitory concentrations [24, 26]. It is approved for the temporary prevention of ocular itching due to allergic conjunctivitis. It is now available as an over-the-counter anti-allergic agent. It has been reported that ketotifen can cause a mild stinging or burning effect on the conjunctiva surface upon instillation [24].

Epinastine 0.05% ophthalmic solution is an antihistamine with mast cell stabilizing and anti-inflammatory properties. It has affinity for H1 and H2 receptors with prolonged therapeutic effect lasting up to 12 hours and onset of action within 3 minutes [41, 42]. Epinastine could inhibit antigen-induced uptake of calcium ion, which in turn, results in the suppression of angiogenic factor synthesis by mast cells. Furthermore, epinastine could inhibit the activation of the transcription factor NF-κB that regulates FcεRI-mediated expression of TNF-α, IL-6 and IL-8 transcripts in mast cells [26, 43]. It is of note that NF-κB, a ubiquitous protein transcription factor, resides in an inactive state in the cytoplasm but upon activation, it translocates to the nucleus where it binds the DNA and activates the expression of inflammatory genes [43]. The anti-inflammatory properties of epinastine could be attributed to the multimodal therapeutic effect, which includes blockade of histamine receptors, mast cell stabilization, inhibition of vasodilation and vasopermeability, and inhibition of the recruitment of neutrophils and eosinophils into the site of allergic inflammatory reaction [41]. Epinastine is a well-tolerated multimodal anti-allergic agent that is dosed twice daily for the prevention of itching associated with allergic conjunctivitis [44]. Because of its neutral pH and neutral impact on the ocular surface, the prolonged use of epinastine during the allergy season could be well-tolerated. It has an excellent safety profile with minimal systemic absorption after topical administration. The most frequently reported ocular adverse effect of epinastine is transient, mild burning sensation in the eye following topical administration [41].

Alcaftadine 0.25% ophthalmic solution, a tricyclic piperidine aldehyde, is a potent histamine receptor antagonist with high affinity for histamine H1 and H2 receptors and a lower affinity for H4 receptors [45, 46]. It also exhibits modulatory action on immune cell recruitment and mast cell stabilizing effects [45]. The ability of alcaftadine to inhibit eosinophil recruitment could be attributed to its binding to H4 receptors, as H4 receptors are expressed on mast cells and leukocytes [45, 47, 48]. The anti-allergic and anti-inflammatory properties of alcaftadine are likely due to its ability to stabilize and protect the tight junction proteins of the conjunctival epithelium from allergic inflammation-induced degradation by proteolytic enzymes secreted by allergens as well as eosinophil-derived epitheliotoxic mediators [45, 47]. Clinical studies have demonstrated the safety and clinical efficacy of once-a-day dosed alcaftadine 0.25% ophthalmic solution, which is approved for the prevention of itching associated with allergic conjunctivitis in patients over 2 years of age [45, 46]. The most frequent side effect associated with the use of alcaftadine are eye irritation, burning and/or stinging upon instillation [45].

Bepotastine besilate 1.5% ophthalmic solution, a piperidine derivative, is a twice-a-day dosed anti-allergic agent with H1-receptor antagonism that is FDA approved for treating itching associated with allergic conjunctivitis in adults and children of 3 years of age and older [49]. Additionally it suppresses eosinophil activation and stabilizes mast cells. The anti-inflammatory property of bepotastine besilate is attributed to its ability to inhibit the production of interleukin-5, a cytokine that plays a role in the activation and survival of eosinophil. Additionally, it suppresses the expression of ICAM-1 required for the accumulation of immune cells at the site of allergic inflammatory reaction, as well as inhibits PAF-induced conjunctival eosinophil infiltration [50]. The most frequent ocular adverse events associated with the use of Bepotastine besilate in approximately 25% of patients are eye irritation and mild abnormal taste following instillation [49].

Nonsteroidal Anti-Inflammatory Drugs

Nonsteroidal Anti-Inflammatory Drugs (NSAID) may be useful, as an adjunct, in treating ocular allergy, as they are effective in relieving pruritus and reducing conjunctival hyperemia. It has been shown that PGE2 and PGI2 act to lower the threshold of conjunctiva to histamine-induced itching. NSAID may be considered a valuable steroid-sparing therapeutic agent since they do not mask ocular infections, affect wound healing, increase intraocular pressure or contribute to the formation of cataracts [1]. Topical formulations, such as ketorolac 0.5% and diclofenac 0.1% have been shown to diminish ocular pruritus and conjunctival hyperemia associated with allergic conjunctivitis. The disadvantage of using these preparations is that they have weaker anti-inflammatory action than topical steroidal agents. While these medications reduce conjunctival hyperemia, they have little effect on papillary size [15]. Bromfenac 0.09% ophthalmic solution is a potent inhibitor of the COX-2 enzyme and highly lipophilic molecule that rapidly penetrates ocular tissues, which in turn, results in an increased duration of action and enhanced therapeutic effect [51]. It blocks the conversion of arachidonic acid into eicosanoids, thus, it prevents vasodilation, pruritus, eosinophil infiltration, and increased conjunctival microvascular permeability induced by PGD2 and PGE2 [52]. Bromfenac 0.09% ophthalmic solution, usually dosed twice a day, is a safe and well-tolerated topical NSAID that downregulates COX-2, an enzyme that mediates ocular inflammation [51]. Because PGD2 and PGE2 are all ocular surface pruritogens, a COX-2 inhibitor may be beneficial in suppressing the pruritogenic and proinflammatory activities of PGs in the conjunctiva [53]. The use of NSAID in the treatment of ocular allergy is limited due to the availability of potent multimodal anti-allergic agents. Although there may be limited concern over the phenomenon of NSAID-induced asthma (topically or orally), it seems to only be a problem in patients who have the triad of asthma, nasal polyposis and aspirin sensitivity [1, 29].

Corticosteroids

Corticosteroids possess potent anti-inflammatory, immunosuppressive and anti-proliferative properties. They inhibit the expression of cytokines, chemokines and adhesion molecules [54], which in turn, results in suppression of cellular infiltration, capillary dilation, fibroblast proliferation, collagen deposition and scar formation. Additionally, corticosteroids will stabilize intracellular and extracellular membranes; increase the synthesis of lipocortins that block phospholipase A2 an enzyme necessary for the hydrolysis of arachidonic acid, this in turn results in reduced production of late-phase allergic inflammatory mediators such as prostaglandins and leukotrienes; and increase the enzyme histaminases that degrades histamine, thereby reducing the amount of unbound histamine on the ocular surface [55]. Although corticosteroids are incapable of blocking histamine receptors, they can inhibit histamine production in mast cells by blocking the action of histidine decarboxylase. Corticosteroids are not effective in stabilizing mast cells due to their inability to prevent calcium influx into the mast cell. Furthermore, corticosteroids can also inhibit neovascularization and reduce capillary permeability [2, 56-58]. Following administration, corticosteroids diffuse readily across cell membranes and enter the cytoplasm, where it undergoes metabolism by 11β - hydroxysteroid dehydrogenase (11β-HSDs) [59]. The glucocorticoid binds to glucocorticoid receptor (GRα) in the cytoplasm to form the GR–corticosteroid complex, with subsequent transportation of the activated GR–corticosteroid complex into the nucleus, where it binds to DNA at specific sequences in the promoter region of corticosteroid-responsive genes (glucocorticoid response elements (GRE)) [54, 60]. The interaction between GR–corticosteroid complex and GRE leads to increased gene transcription (transactivation process) characterized by activation of genes encoding anti-inflammatory mediators, such as secretory leukoprotease inhibitor (SLPI), mitogen-activated protein kinase phosphatase-1 (MKP-1), annexin-1 (lipocortin-1), inhibitor of nuclear factor κB (IκB-α) and glucocorticoid-induced leucine zipper (GILZ) [60, 61]. Infrequently, GR interacts with negative GRE leading to repression of gene transcription (cis-repression) characterized by reduction in keratin, osteocalcin, and corticotrophin releasing factor. The GR–corticosteroid complex in the nucleus also interacts with co-activator molecules such as CREB (cyclic AMP response element-binding protein)-binding protein (CREBBP or CBP)) that are activated by pro-inflammatory transcription factors (e.g. AP-1 and NF-κB). This interaction suppresses the effects of proinflammatory transcription factors (transrepression) that regulate the expression of inflammatory genes that code for many inflammatory proteins, such as cytokines (IL-2, IL-3, IL-4, IL-5, IL-6, IL-13, IL-15, TNF-α, GM-CSF, TSLP), chemokines (CCL1, CCL5, CCL11, CXCL8), inflammatory enzymes, adhesion molecules (ICAM-1,VCAM-1) and inflammatory receptors [61]. Thus, through transrepression, GR–corticosteroid complex modulates the transcription rates of non-GRE-containing genes by interacting with nuclear transcription factors [59].

Corticosteroids play a major role in the treatment of ocular allergic diseases, since it can hinder the transcription factor GATA-3 that regulates the transcription of Th2-derived cytokine genes and differentiation of activated T-lymphocytes into Th2-lymphocytes. This immunosuppressive effect is accomplished by corticosteroid-induced increase in expression of MAPK phosphatase-1 (MKP-1) that inhibits p38 MAPK (mitogen-activated protein kinase)-mediated phosphorylation of GATA3. The phosphorylation of GATA-3 is necessary for interaction with importin-α, a nuclear transporter protein necessary for translocation of GATA-3 into the nucleus [61, 62]. Additionally, the corticosteroid-activated GR competes with activated GATA-3 for importin-α, a nuclear transporter protein that plays a role in the nuclear transport of GR [61, 62]. Proinflammatory transcription factors, such as NF-κB and activator protein-1 (AP-1) are activated in all inflammatory ocular surface diseases and play a major role in amplifying and perpetuating the inflammatory process in allergic disorders. The major effect of corticosteroid in controlling allergic inflammation is to deactivate the inflammatory genes that are involved in encoding cytokines, chemokines, adhesion molecules, inflammatory enzymes, receptors and proteins that interact and activate structural cells at the site of allergic inflammatory reaction [60].

Loteprednol etabonate ophthalmic suspension, a cortienic acid-based derivative, is a highly lipophilic anti-inflammatory agent with enhanced penetrability through biological membranes. Following topical administration, the drug becomes highly concentrated in the cornea (primary site of metabolism) followed by the iris/ciliary body and aqueous humor [55]. Loteprednol is more lipophilic than ketone corticosteroids such as prednisolone, and as such, the highly lipophilic nature of this anti-inflammatory agent may contribute to its increased efficacy by enhancing penetration into target cells [63]. Loteprednol etabonate ophthalmic suspension, a site-specific soft steroid, primarily targets the late phase inflammatory aspect of the ocular allergic response. It is site specific in view of the fact that the active drug resides at the site of allergic inflammation long enough to render its therapeutic effect without causing adverse drug reactions, such as raised intraocular pressure (IOP) and cataract [4, 58, 63]. The long-term use of loteprednol is likely to have a lower propensity to induce IOP elevation even when used in known steroid responders since its active form undergoes rapid transformation into an inactive carboxylic acid metabolite (cortienic acid). This rapid transformation reduces the possibility of toxicity and duration of exposure of the anterior segment including the anterior chamber to the active form of loteprednol. This rapid transformation at the site of inflammation after rendering its therapeutic effect is due to the effect of numerous esterases in the eye. Loteprednol, unlike ketone corticosteroids that have the ketone group at C-20 position, rarely causes cataract formation, as it is unable to form a covalent bond with lens protein that could result in cataractogenesis. However, the presence of other mechanisms that can induce cataractogenesis cannot be ruled out [55]. Additionally, adverse drug reactions such as cataract formation and IOP elevation are minimized due to its retrometabolic design, as loteprednol etabonate meets the required balance between solubility/lipophilicity, ocular tissue distribution, GR receptor binding, and metabolic deactivation to inactive metabolites after exerting their desired therapeutic effect, all of which are essential features of retrometabolic drug design [55]. Loteprednol is a suitable long-term therapeutic option for chronic ocular allergies due to their superior safety profile relative to the ketone corticosteroids [2, 31, 58, 63]. It has been demonstrated to be effective in treating allergic conjunctivitis and giant papillary conjunctivitis [3]. Loteprednol etabonate was shown to be safe and effective when used for 12 months or more for the treatment of seasonal or perennial allergic conjunctivitis [58].

Rimexoline (a derivative of prednisolone) is quickly inactivated in the anterior chamber of the eye, thus leading to improved efficacy and decreased safety concerns [1].

Prednisolone acetate 1.0% is a an excellent choice for treating severe inflammatory disorders due to its good ocular penetrability while prednisolone sodium phosphate (0.125% and 1.0%) may be considered a suitable drug for moderate inflammatory disorders of the ocular surface due to its reduced ocular penetrability when compared to prednisolone acetate [64]. When corticosteroids with lower potency are ineffective, more potent steroids (prednisolone, dexamethasone, betamethasone) can be employed [1].

Fluorometholone (21- deoxy-9-fluoro-6-methyl presnisolone) is an anti-inflammatory steroid with an anti-inflammatory activity 25 to 30 times that of hydrocortisone [65]. The fluorometholone-based steroids are used for treating mild to moderate ocular surface inflammatory conditions and chronic inflammatory condition requiring prolonged steroidal therapy. They have reduced propensity to induce an IOP rise. The acetate form of fluorometholone-based steroids has greater anti-inflammatory activity than the alcohol form due to their enhanced bioavailability [64]. Clinical studies have shown that fluorometholone-based steroids reduces the clinical expression of VKC, including discharge, conjunctival redness, papillary hypertrophy and Horners Tranta's dots [3, 20].

Cream-based steroid such as triamcinolone and hydrocortisone are useful for treating periocular inflammation in contact ocular allergy [64].

Topical corticosteroids are potent anti-allergic agents that are considered appropriate for the treatment of chronic ocular allergic conditions, as they have the ability to suppress the recruitment and activation of pro-inflammatory allergic mediators during ocular allergic response [22, 64]. Topical mast cell stabilizers are less effective in controlling the acute exacerbations seen in T-lymphocyte-mediated chronic ocular allergy. Topical corticosteroids are the T-cell-targeted therapeutic agents that are beneficial in treating allergic eye diseases such as VKC and AKC, in which T-cell infiltration is a prominent feature. Topical steroidal therapy is likely to be useful in cases of ocular surface damage caused by the release of epithelial toxic mediators from eosinophils and neutrophils. It is advisable to start with steroids with low absorption and enhanced therapeutic index (e.g., loteprednol) with the dosing being based on the state of inflammation of the ocular surface. Rimexolone

1.0% and loteprednol (0.2% and 0.5%) are two modified corticosteroids with low absorption and improved efficacy [1].

Topical ophthalmic corticosteroids can cause adverse reactions such as elevations in IOP, cataract formation following extended use, delayed wound healing, and lower resistance to infection [55]. Most side effects of corticosteroids appear to be due to DNA binding and gene activation (cis-repression). To minimize these adverse effects, topical steroids with potent trans-repression with relatively little trans-activation or cis-repression activity (dissociated steroid) [60] are preferred and they may become the corticosteroid of choice for treating chronic ocular allergies. It is of note that fluticasone propionate and budesonide, topical steroids used in asthma therapy appear to have more potent trans-repression than trans-activation effects, thus reducing the potential risk of systemic side effects [60].

Immunomodulators

Immunomodulators, such as cyclosporine and tacrolimus, play vital roles in the treatment of allergic eye diseases due to their ability to inhibit calcineurin, a protein phosphatase that is essential in activating transcription factors required for IL-2 production, an important activator of T-lymphocyte activation [66, 67]. Immunomodulators are known to inhibit FcεRI-mediated release of preformed and newly formed mediators from mast cells [3]. Additionally, they are capable of blocking mast cell proliferation, blocking release of cytokines from T-lymphocytes, and reducing eosinophil chemotaxis [20].

Tacrolimus, a potent macrolide immunosuppressor, exerts its action by inhibiting IgE production by activated B-cells, as well as preventing T-cell activation and associated pro-inflammatory cytokine production. Tacrolimus also interferes with mast cell degranulation; suppresses antigen presentation by down-regulating FcεRI in Langerhans' cells; and suppressing late phase responses in ocular allergy. Tacrolimus could be therapeutically beneficial for patients with atopic keratoconjunctivitis (AKC), vernal keratoconjunctivitis, atopic eyelid disease and atopic dermatitis [1, 66, 68-70]. Tacrolimus ointment is recommended for maintenance therapy and induction therapy [71]. Tacrolimus (0.1 and 0.03%) has been approved for topical use in atopic dermatitis [1]. Tacrolimus is considered to be a safe and well-tolerated drug for long-term management of atopic dermatitis, as it does not cause skin atrophy, telangiectasia or increased intraocular pressure [71, 72]. Drug concentrations in the systemic circulation are low with topical use [70]. Tacrolimus ointment, unlike steroids, does not reduce collagen synthesis, and as such, it can be used safely on the face and neck [73] for treating atopic dermatitis that is unresponsive to topical corticosteroids [71]. Although there are concerns such as potential to be carcinogenic regarding the topical use of tacrolimus [1], such concerns is with regards to using topical immunomodulators in treating atopic dermatitis in children, rather than chronic contact dermatitis in adults [74]. Application of tacrolimus can cause transient burning sensation and hot flashes to the applied area, as well as induce local immune suppression with the attendant risk of increasing a patient's susceptibility to local infections and recurrent herpetic lesions [71, 75]. Additional side effects of tacrolimus include pancytopenia, hyperglycemia, hyperkalemia, tremor, headache, insomnia, hypertension, dyspnea, pleural effusion, diarrhea, nausea and vomiting, pruritus, muscle cramps, nephropathy and arthalgia [72].

Cyclosporine (CsA) is a cyclic undecapeptide produced by the fungi Tolypocladium inflatum and Beauveria nevus [66]. Cyclosporine exerts its immunosuppressive action by binding to a cyclophilin to form a cyclosporine-cyclophilin A complex that inhibits the activity of the calcineurin phosphatase, an enzyme involved in immunological signaling pathway. Cyclosporine-mediated inhibition of calcineurin blocks dephosphorylation of NFAT in the cytoplasm, thereby preventing its translocation to the nucleus, where it is needed to induce the transcription of several cytokine genes, such as IL-2 involved in T-cell activation [66, 67, 72]. Because CsA exerts its immunosuppressive effect by blocking IL-2 production and Th2-lymphocyte proliferation, it should be quite effective in controlling ocular inflammation. Additional anti-inflammatory effects of CsA are demonstrated by its ability to inhibit histamine release from mast cells and reduce eosinophil chemotaxis via inhibition of IL-5 production. It is also beneficial in treating patients with Th1-lymphocyte-mediated DTH, as it inhibits IFN-γ production [76]. Cyclosporine is prescribed, when steroids are contraindicated or unsafe, for treating the severe form or steroid resistant cases of chronic ocular allergy [3]. A clinical study found 0.05% cyclosporin A, dosed 4 − 6 times daily was effective in alleviating signs and symptoms of severe AKC refractory to topical steroid treatment [1]. Additionally, it has been shown that topical CsA 0.05% had a significant beneficial effect on patients with VKC and AKC [76]. Because of the efficacy and tolerability of CsA in AD, it is used as the second-choice therapy in patients with severe, recalcitrant AD who cannot be controlled with standard topical therapy [67, 72]. CsA exhibits its strong anti-pruritic effect by suppressing T-cell derived pruritic mediators such as IL-2 and probably IL-31, and as such, it could be useful in controlling the inflammatory skin condition in patients with AD [72].

Anti-Metabolites

Mitomycin-C, an antimetabolite, selectively inhibits DNA synthesis and is non–cell-cycle specific but at high concentrations, it could suppress cellular RNA and protein production [77]. It is a non-selective inhibitor of the migration and proliferation of inflammatory cells and fibroblasts [78]. The mitomycin-C induced inhibition of DNA synthesis hinders cell migration and mitosis, which in turn, results in a decreased rate of cell proliferation [77]. Thus, mitomycin-C should be used with caution in patients with corneal epithelial defects, as inhibition of cell proliferation would delay the corneal wound repair process. Mitomycin-C has been shown to inhibit regrowth of corneal pannus after surgical excision in patients with atopic keratoconjunctivitis [77]. Mitomycin C (MMC) 0.01% eye drops have been shown to decrease mucous discharge, conjunctival hyperemia and limbal edema in patients with VKC [15]. Jain and colleagues recommended the use of 0.01% MMC eye drops in patients with recalcitrant and severe cases of VKC that were unresponsive to topical steroid and mast cell stabilizers [78]. Sodhi et al [79] demonstrated that low dose topical MMC was effective in the treatment of allergic conjunctivitis.

Allergen Specific Immunotherapy

Current therapies for allergic eye diseases include non-pharmacological modalities such as allergen avoidance, administration of preservative-free ocular lubricants in their cold state to dilute and flush away allergens, and cool compresses to induce vasoconstriction [80]. Pharmacological therapy includes antihistamines, mast cell stabilizers, multimodal action anti-allergic, and anti-inflammatory pharmaceutical agents.

Allergen-specific immunotherapy is based on the principle that exposure to allergens not only provokes allergic inflammation but also induces immunological tolerance. Allergen-specific immunotherapy (SIT) that involves the administration of gradually increasing amounts of an allergen extract has been used successfully to treat mild asthma and allergic rhinitis [72].

Allergen-specific immunotherapy is an effective treatment used by allergists and immunologists for patients with allergic rhinoconjunctivitis and/or allergic asthma. Additionally, it is indicated for patients with allergic clinical expressions that are not well controlled with non-pharmacological and pharmacological therapeutic modalities; require high doses of medication and/or multiple medications to maintain control of their allergic disease; or experience adverse effects of medications [81].

The primary goal of allergen-specific immunotherapy is to decrease the clinical expression of allergic diseases and prevent recurrence of the disease by inducing allergen-specific clinical tolerance to the offending allergen [81, 82]. It is of note that for allergen-specific immunotherapy to be effective, the patient must have a history of developing clinical features of allergy when exposed to the offending allergen, as well as evidence of IgE antibodies to the specific allergen as demonstrated by skin prick test or radioallergosorbent test [82].

Subcutaneous immunotherapy (SCIT) involves the subcutaneous administration of gradually increasing quantities of the relevant allergens until a dose is reached that is effective in inducing immunologic tolerance to the allergens. The SCIT induces a shift from Th2-lymphocyte immune responses, which is associated with the development of allergic disease, to Th1-lymphocyte immune responses. It is also associated with the production of T-regulatory cells that produce the anti-inflammatory cytokine, IL-10 and TGF-β that downregulates allergen-induced Th2-lymphocyte-mediated immune responses [81, 82]. IL-10 reduces the levels of allergen-specific IgE antibodies and induces the production of allergen-specific IgG4 antibodies that play a role in secondary immune responses. Additionally, IL-10 inhibits the recruitment and activation of mast cells and eosinophils to the eye [81, 83]. TGF-β1 decreases mast cell and eosinophil activation and induces immunoglobulin class switching toward IgG and IgA and away from IgE [83]. Thus, allergen-specific immunotherapy reduces the recruitment of mast cells and eosinophils to the eye after exposure to allergens and reduces the release of mediators from mast cells [81].

Sublingual immunotherapy (SLIT) is an oral form of allergen-specific immunotherapy administered as soluble tablets or drops to be kept under the tongue for 1–2 min and then swallowed. SLIT is usually administered either prior to the spring or fall pollen allergy season to prevent clinical expression induced by seasonal allergens, or continuously throughout the year to prevent symptoms from perennial allergens [82]. Following administration, oral mucosal Langerhans bound with SLIT allergen migrate to regional lymph nodes, where they interact with naïve T-lymphocytes resulting in the generation of allergen-specific regulatory T lymphocytes [83]. SLIT induces a dose- and time-dependent increase in the production of tolerogenic cytokines (IL-10 and TGF-β1), which in turn, results in an attenuation of seasonal increases in allergen-specific IgE levels, as well as time- and dose-dependent increase in allergen-specific IgG4 and IgA [82, 83]. SLIT can also induce the production of allergen-specific IFN-γ production that dampens Th2-lymphocyte-mediated immune response. SLIT has been demonstrated to reduce the levels of conjunctival eosinophils, neutrophils, and expression of intracellular adhesion molecule-1 [83].

Local conjunctival immunotherapy (LCIT) is another type of allergen-specific immunotherapy, for treating allergic conjunctivitis. It involves the administration of an eye drop containing specific allergens into the conjunctiva, which in turn, results in inducing an increased tolerance to the offending allergen and control of the allergic expression in the eye without relying on anti-allergic pharmacotherapy. This mode of allergen-specific immunotherapy is safe and well tolerated and is very beneficial for patients with perennial allergic conjunctivitis [84].

Because the oral microenvironment is regarded as a site of natural immune tolerance, SLIT appears to have a good safety profile with the main side effects being local (oral itching) as opposed to systemic allergic reactions [82, 83]. Patients receiving allergen-specific immunotherapy should be educated on the local and systemic side effects. Local side effects associated with the use of SCIT include redness or itching at the injection site, which can be managed with local treatment (e.g., cool compresses or topical corticosteroids) or oral antihistamines. The systemic side effect of SCIT is usually mild but there is a risk of developing anaphylactic reactions, and as such, allergist or immunologist should only prescribe SCIT. Allergen-specific immunotherapy is generally safe and well-tolerated when used in appropriately selected patients [81].

Although studies have proven the safety and efficacy of allergen-specific immunotherapy (AIT) for the treatment of allergic rhinitis, allergic conjunctivitis and allergic asthma, this treatment modality should be considered for patients who have demonstrated specific IgE antibodies to a relevant allergen or allergens [85].

Practice Management

In the management of ocular allergy, it is imperative to categorize the severity of the condition into mild, moderate or severe. This will aid in educating the patient and/or their parent on the duration of the treatment, the treatment itself, long-term management plan and prognosis [86]. The clinician is responsible for educating the patient on the nature of their allergic disease process; the different modalities for managing ocular allergy; the need for long-term management; and the correct way of applying topical anti-allergy medication. Additionally, adequate knowledge of anti-allergic and anti-inflammatory pharmaceutical agents used in the management of allergic eye diseases is necessary. It is important for clinicians to familiarize themselves with the different types of anti-allergic and anti-inflammatory medications, their mode of action, their indications, side-effect profile, contra-indications, and relative efficacies. A clinician who has proficient knowledge of these factors will be in a good position to prescribe the appropriate type of anti-allergy and/or anti-inflammatory medication that will best address the allergic reaction [80].

The mainstay of the management of ocular allergy involves the use of anti-allergic therapeutic agents such as antihistamine, multmodal anti-allergic agents and mast cell stabilizers. When anti-allergic therapeutic agents are incapable of providing adequate therapeutic effect or control of the allergic inflammatory process, the clinician should prescribe an anti-inflammatory agent. Topical immunomodulators such as tacrolimus are steroid-free alternatives that could be beneficial when long-term use of topical steroids is not a safe therapeutic option. The once-a-day or twice-a-day dosed multmodal anti-allergic agents have prophylactic and therapeutic properties, and as such, they may be considered the preferred choice for managing allergic conjunctivitis. Mast cell stabilizing drugs are an excellent choice for long-term prophylactic and maintenance therapy in patients with recurrent and perennial ocular allergy [3]. When a clinician decides to use a steroid to control hyperacute or chronic ocular allergic expressions, the topical steroid with an excellent safety profile and suitable for prolonged use such as loteprednol etabonate may be used as the drug of choice. Other suitable topical steroids are rimexolone, prednisolone and fluorometholone [63].

Knowledge of the patient's life style is helpful in promoting compliance with recommended treatment protocols. To promote patient compliance, the clinician could prescribe anti-allergic and/or anti-inflammatory therapeutic agents that provide a rapid clinical response and prolonged therapeutic effect.

Furthermore, prescribing therapeutic agents that are cost-effective and comfortable with less frequent dosing and good safety profile, will also enhance compliance. Individuals with busy lifestyles such as students and workers may benefit from using once-a-day or twice-a-day dosed, long-acting topical anti-allergic agents. Agents such as these will improve compliance and avoid the issue of self-administration in the case of young school-aged children. Once-daily dosed anti-allergic therapeutic agents may be considered the therapeutic agent of choice for school-aged children due to their convenience of use. If a patient complains of stinging or burning effect of the topical medication, in order to ensure compliance, the clinician could advise the patient to keep them in the refrigerator and apply them to the eye in the cold state. This non-pharmacologic management strategy will promote compliance with recommended treatment protocol [80].

In acute ocular allergy, the use of anti-allergic medications along with supportive therapy is usually sufficient. In hyperacute cases and chronic ocular allergy, it is preferable to control the inflammatory condition with an anti-inflammatory agent, such as steroids, for short-term therapy and a multimodal anti-allergic agent for long-term therapy. Thus, pulse steroidal therapy would become necessary if the allergic expression does not respond to anti-allergic therapy. The correct management of ocular allergy is imperative to avoid an adverse effect on the patient's quality of life, as well as the ocular surface damage that might occur if this condition is under-treated or left untreated [80].

References

[1]   Manzouri, B., et al., Pharmacotherapy of allergic eye disease. *Expert Opin Pharmacother,* 2006. 7(9): p. 1191-200.

[2]   Bielory, L., Ocular allergy treatment. *Immunol Allergy Clin North Am,* 2008. 28(1): p. 189-224, vii.

[3]   Leonardi, A., Emerging drugs for ocular allergy. *Expert Opin Emerg Drugs,* 2005. 10(3): p. 505-20.

[4]   Bielory, L., Ocular allergy overview. *Immunol Allergy Clin North Am,* 2008. 28(1): p. 1-23, v.

[5]   Abelson, M. and J. Greiner, Comparative efficacy of olopatadine 0.1% ophthalmic solution versus levocabastine 0.05% ophthalmic suspension using the conjunctival allergen challenge model. *Curr Med Res Opin,* 2004. 20(12): p. 1953-8.

[6] Bielory, L., et al., Treating the ocular component of allergic rhinoconjunctivitis and related eye disorders. *MedGenMed*, 2007. 9(3): p. 35.

[7] Inomata, N., S. Tatewaki, and Z. Ikezawa, Multiple H1-antihistamine-induced urticaria. *J Dermatol*, 2009. 36(4): p. 224-7.

[8] Campoli-Richards, D.M., M.M. Buckley, and A. Fitton, Cetirizine. A review of its pharmacological properties and clinical potential in allergic rhinitis, pollen-induced asthma, and chronic urticaria. *Drugs*, 1990. 40(5): p. 762-81.

[9] Bonini, S., et al., The eosinophil and the eye. *Allergy*, 1997. 52(34 Suppl): p. 44-7.

[10] Dockhorn, R.J., et al., Safety and efficacy of loratadine (Sch-29851): a new non-sedating antihistamine in seasonal allergic rhinitis. *Ann Allergy*, 1987. 58(6): p. 407-11.

[11] Barenholtz, H.A. and D.C. McLeod, Loratadine: a nonsedating antihistamine with once-daily dosing. *DICP*, 1989. 23(6): p. 445-50.

[12] Eda, R., et al., Effect of loratadine on human eosinophil function in vitro. *Ann Allergy*, 1993. 71(4): p. 373-8.

[13] Clissold, S.P., E.M. Sorkin, and K.L. Goa, Loratadine. A preliminary review of its pharmacodynamic properties and therapeutic efficacy. *Drugs*, 1989. 37(1): p. 42-57.

[14] Noble, S. and D. McTavish, Levocabastine. An update of its pharmacology, clinical efficacy and tolerability in the topical treatment of allergic rhinitis and conjunctivitis. *Drugs*, 1995. 50(6): p. 1032-49.

[15] Kumar, S., Vernal keratoconjunctivitis: a major review. *Acta Ophthalmol*, 2009. 87(2): p. 133-47.

[16] Yanni, J., et al., Inhibition of histamine-induced human conjunctival epithelial cell responses by ocular allergy drugs. *Arch Ophthalmol*, 1999. 117(5): p. 643-7.

[17] Discepola, M., J. Deschenes, and M. Abelson, Comparison of the topical ocular antiallergic efficacy of emedastine 0.05% ophthalmic solution to ketorolac 0.5% ophthalmic solution in a clinical model of allergic conjunctivitis. *Acta Ophthalmol Scand Suppl*, 1999(228): p. 43-6.

[18] Horak, F., et al., Onset and duration of action of ketotifen 0.025% and emedastine 0.05% in seasonal allergic conjunctivitis : efficacy after repeated pollen challenges in the vienna challenge chamber. *Clin Drug Investig*, 2003. 23(5): p. 329-37.

[19] D'Arienzo, P., A. Leonardi, and G. Bensch, Randomized, double-masked, placebo-controlled comparison of the efficacy of emedastine

difumarate 0.05% ophthalmic solution and ketotifen fumarate 0.025% ophthalmic solution in the human conjunctival allergen challenge model. *Clin Ther,* 2002. 24(3): p. 409-16.

[20] Abelson, M., L. Smith, and M. Chapin, Ocular allergic disease: mechanisms, disease sub-types, treatment. *Ocul Surf,* 2003. 1(3): p. 127-49.

[21] Katelaris, C., et al., A comparison of the efficacy and tolerability of olopatadine hydrochloride 0.1% ophthalmic solution and cromolyn sodium 2% ophthalmic solution in seasonal allergic conjunctivitis. *Clin Ther,* 2002. 24(10): p. 1561-75.

[22] Leonardi, A., The central role of conjunctival mast cells in the pathogenesis of ocular allergy. *Curr Allergy Asthma Rep,* 2002. 2(4): p. 325-31.

[23] Bonini, S., A. Lambiase, and R. Sgrulletta, Allergic chronic inflammation of the ocular surface in vernal keratoconjunctivitis. *Curr Opin Allergy Clin Immunol,* 2003. 3(5): p. 381-7.

[24] Bielory, L., Ocular allergy guidelines: a practical treatment algorithm. *Drugs,* 2002. 62(11): p. 1611-34.

[25] Leonardi, A. and A.G. Secchi, Vernal keratoconjunctivitis. *Int Ophthalmol Clin,* 2003. 43(1): p. 41-58.

[26] Lambiase, A., A. Micera, and S. Bonini, Multiple action agents and the eye: do they really stabilize mast cells? *Curr Opin Allergy Clin Immunol,* 2009. 9(5): p. 454-65.

[27] Solomon, A., J. Pe'er, and F. Levi-Schaffer, Advances in ocular allergy: basic mechanisms, clinical patterns and new therapies. *Curr Opin Allergy Clin Immunol,* 2001. 1(5): p. 477-82.

[28] Alexander, M., S. Allegro, and A. Hicks, Efficacy and acceptability of nedocromil sodium 2% and olopatadine hydrochloride 0.1% in perennial allergic conjunctivitis. *Adv Ther.* 17(3): p. 140-7.

[29] Verin, P., Treating severe eye allergy. *Clin Exp Allergy,* 1998. 28 Suppl 6: p. 44-8.

[30] Abelson, M., et al., Efficacy of olopatadine ophthalmic solution 0.2% in reducing signs and symptoms of allergic conjunctivitis. *Allergy Asthma Proc.* 28(4): p. 427-33.

[31] Berdy, G., J. Stoppel, and A. Epstein, Comparison of the clinical efficacy and tolerability of olopatadine hydrochloride 0.1% ophthalmic solution and loteprednol etabonate 0.2% ophthalmic suspension in the conjunctival allergen challenge model. *Clin Ther,* 2002. 24(6): p. 918-29.

[32] Deschenes, J., M. Discepola, and M. Abelson, Comparative evaluation of olopatadine ophthalmic solution (0.1%) versus ketorolac ophthalmic solution (0.5%) using the provocative antigen challenge model. *Acta Ophthalmol Scand Suppl,* 1999(228): p. 47-52.

[33] Abelson, M. and P. Gomes, Olopatadine 0.2% ophthalmic solution: the first ophthalmic antiallergy agent with once-daily dosing. *Expert Opin Drug Metab Toxicol,* 2008. 4(4): p. 453-61.

[34] Bielory, L., P. Buddiga, and S. Bigelson, Ocular allergy treatment comparisons: azelastine and olopatadine. *Curr Allergy Asthma Rep,* 2004. 4(4): p. 320-5.

[35] Corum, I., et al., Efficiency of olopatadine hydrochloride 0.1% in the treatment of vernal keratoconjunctivitis and goblet cell density. *J Ocul Pharmacol Ther,* 2005. 21(5): p. 400-5.

[36] Ciprandi, G., G. Passalacqua, and G.W. Canonica, Effects of H1 antihistamines on adhesion molecules: a possible rationale for long-term treatment. *Clin Exp Allergy,* 1999. 29 Suppl 3: p. 49-53.

[37] Ciprandi, G., et al., Azelastine eye drops reduce and prevent allergic conjunctival reaction and exert anti-allergic activity. *Clin Exp Allergy,* 1997. 27(2): p. 182-91.

[38] Spangler, D., G. Bensch, and G. Berdy, Evaluation of the efficacy of olopatadine hydrochloride 0.1% ophthalmic solution and azelastine hydrochloride 0.05% ophthalmic solution in the conjunctival allergen challenge model. *Clin Ther,* 2001. 23(8): p. 1272-80.

[39] Giede, C., et al., Comparison of azelastine eye drops with levocabastine eye drops in the treatment of seasonal allergic conjunctivitis. *Curr Med Res Opin,* 2000. 16(3): p. 153-63.

[40] Greiner, J., et al., Single dose of ketotifen fumarate .025% vs 2 weeks of cromolyn sodium 4% for allergic conjunctivitis. *Adv Ther.* 19(4): p. 185-93.

[41] Trattler, W., J. Luchs, and P. Majmudar, Elestat (epinastine HCl ophthalmic solution 0.05%) as a therapeutic for allergic conjunctivitis. *Int Ophthalmol Clin,* 2006. 46(4): p. 87-99.

[42] Friedlaender, M., Epinastine in the management of ocular allergic disease. *Int Ophthalmol Clin,* 2006. 46(4): p. 85-6.

[43] Asano, K., et al., Inhibition of angiogenic factor production from murine mast cells by an antiallergic agent (epinastine hydrochloride) in vitro. *Mediators Inflamm,* 2008. 2008: p. 265095.

[44] Borazan, M., et al., Efficacy of olopatadine HCI 0.1%, ketotifen fumarate 0.025%, epinastine HCI 0.05%, emedastine 0.05% and

fluorometholone acetate 0.1% ophthalmic solutions for seasonal allergic conjunctivitis: a placebo-controlled environmental trial. *Acta Ophthalmol,* 2009. 87(5): p. 549-54.

[45] Namdar, R. and C. Valdez, Alcaftadine: a topical antihistamine for use in allergic conjunctivitis. *Drugs Today* (Barc), 2011. 47(12): p. 883-90.

[46] Bohets, H., et al., Clinical pharmacology of alcaftadine, a novel antihistamine for the prevention of allergic conjunctivitis. *J Ocul Pharmacol Ther,* 2011. 27(2): p. 187-95.

[47] Ono, S.J. and K. Lane, Comparison of effects of alcaftadine and olopatadine on conjunctival epithelium and eosinophil recruitment in a murine model of allergic conjunctivitis. *Drug Des Devel Ther,* 2011. 5: p. 74-84.

[48] Greiner, J.V., K. Edwards-Swanson, and A. Ingerman, Evaluation of alcaftadine 0.25% ophthalmic solution in acute allergic conjunctivitis at 15 minutes and 16 hours after instillation versus placebo and olopatadine 0.1%. *Clin Ophthalmol,* 2011. 5: p. 87-93.

[49] Wingard, J.B. and F.S. Mah, Critical appraisal of bepotastine in the treatment of ocular itching associated with allergic conjunctivitis. *Clin Ophthalmol,* 2011. 5: p. 201-7.

[50] Kida, T., et al., Bepotastine besilate, a highly selective histamine H(1) receptor antagonist, suppresses vascular hyperpermeability and eosinophil recruitment in in vitro and in vivo experimental allergic conjunctivitis models. *Exp Eye Res,* 2010. 91(1): p. 85-91.

[51] Cho, H., K.J. Wolf, and E.J. Wolf, Management of ocular inflammation and pain following cataract surgery: focus on bromfenac ophthalmic solution. *Clin Ophthalmol,* 2009. 3: p. 199-210.

[52] Hashimoto, T., et al., Effects of nonsteroidal anti-inflammatory drugs on experimental allergic conjunctivitis in Guinea pigs. *J Ocul Pharmacol Ther,* 2003. 19(6): p. 569-77.

[53] Woodward, D., A. Nieves, and M. Friedlaender, Characterization of receptor subtypes involved in prostanoid-induced conjunctival pruritus and their role in mediating allergic conjunctival itching. *J Pharmacol Exp Ther,* 1996. 279(1): p. 137-42.

[54] Almawi, W.Y. and O.K. Melemedjian, Molecular mechanisms of glucocorticoid antiproliferative effects: antagonism of transcription factor activity by glucocorticoid receptor. *J Leukoc Biol,* 2002. 71(1): p. 9-15.

[55] Comstock, T.L. and H.H. Decory, Advances in corticosteroid therapy for ocular inflammation: loteprednol etabonate. *Int J Inflam,* 2012. 2012: p. 789623.

[56] Butrus, S. and R. Portela, Ocular allergy: diagnosis and treatment. *Ophthalmol Clin North Am,* 2005. 18(4): p. 485-92, v.

[57] Durham, S., The inflammatory nature of allergic disease. *Clin Exp Allergy,* 1998. 28 Suppl 6: p. 20-4.

[58] Ilyas, H., et al., Long-term safety of loteprednol etabonate 0.2% in the treatment of seasonal and perennial allergic conjunctivitis. *Eye Contact Lens,* 2004. 30(1): p. 10-3.

[59] McMaster, A. and D.W. Ray, Modelling the glucocorticoid receptor and producing therapeutic agents with anti-inflammatory effects but reduced side-effects. *Exp Physiol,* 2007. 92(2): p. 299-309.

[60] Barnes, P.J., How corticosteroids control inflammation: Quintiles Prize Lecture 2005. *Br J Pharmacol,* 2006. 148(3): p. 245-54.

[61] Barnes, P.J., Glucocorticosteroids: current and future directions. *Br J Pharmacol,* 2011. 163(1): p. 29-43.

[62] Maneechotesuwan, K., et al., Suppression of GATA-3 nuclear import and phosphorylation: a novel mechanism of corticosteroid action in allergic disease. *PLoS Med,* 2009. 6(5): p. e1000076.

[63] Pavesio, C. and H. Decory, Treatment of ocular inflammatory conditions with loteprednol etabonate. *Br J Ophthalmol,* 2008. 92(4): p. 455-9.

[64] Melton, R. and R. Thomas, Clinical Guide to Ophthalmic Drugs. *Review of Optometry,* 2003. 140(6): p. *Supplement:* 33A -39A.

[65] Morrison, E. and D.B. Archer, Effect of fluorometholone (FML) on the intraocular pressure of corticosteroid responders. *Br J Ophthalmol,* 1984. 68(8): p. 581-4.

[66] Donnenfeld, E. and S. Pflugfelder, Topical ophthalmic cyclosporine: pharmacology and clinical uses. *Surv Ophthalmol.* 54(3): p. 321-38.

[67] Ricci, G., et al., Systemic therapy of atopic dermatitis in children. *Drugs,* 2009. 69(3): p. 297-306.

[68] Cheer, S. and G. Plosker, Tacrolimus ointment. A review of its therapeutic potential as a topical therapy in atopic dermatitis. *Am J Clin Dermatol,* 2001. 2(6): p. 389-406.

[69] Paller, A., et al., Three times weekly tacrolimus ointment reduces relapse in stabilized atopic dermatitis: a new paradigm for use. *Pediatrics,* 2008. 122(6): p. e1210-8.

[70] Katsarou, A., et al., Tacrolimus ointment 0.1% in the treatment of allergic contact eyelid dermatitis. *J Eur Acad Dermatol Venereol,* 2009. 23(4): p. 382-7.

[71] Saeki, H., et al., Guidelines for management of atopic dermatitis. *J Dermatol,* 2009. 36(10): p. 563-77.

[72] Katoh, N., Future perspectives in the treatment of atopic dermatitis. *J Dermatol,* 2009. 36(7): p. 367-76.

[73] Reitamo, S., et al., 0.03% Tacrolimus ointment applied once or twice daily is more efficacious than 1% hydrocortisone acetate in children with moderate to severe atopic dermatitis: results of a randomized double-blind controlled trial. *Br J Dermatol,* 2004. 150(3): p. 554-62.

[74] Jacob, S.E. and M.P. Castanedo-Tardan, Pharmacotherapy for allergic contact dermatitis. *Expert Opin Pharmacother,* 2007. 8(16): p. 2757-74.

[75] Miyazaki, D., et al., Therapeutic effects of tacrolimus ointment for refractory ocular surface inflammatory diseases. *Ophthalmology,* 2008. 115(6): p. 988-992 e5.

[76] Keklikci, U., et al., Efficacy of topical cyclosporin A 0.05% in conjunctival impression cytology specimens and clinical findings of severe vernal keratoconjunctivitis in children. *Jpn J Ophthalmol,* 2008. 52(5): p. 357-62.

[77] Akpek, E., et al., A randomized trial of low-dose, topical mitomycin-C in the treatment of severe vernal keratoconjunctivitis. *Ophthalmology,* 2000. 107(2): p. 263-9.

[78] Jain, A.K. and J. Sukhija, Low dose mitomycin-C in severe vernal keratoconjunctivitis: a randomized prospective double blind study. *Indian J Ophthalmol,* 2006. 54(2): p. 111-6.

[79] Sodhi, P., R. Pandey, and S. Ratan, Efficacy and safety of topical azelastine compared with topical mitomycin C in patients with allergic conjunctivitis. *Cornea,* 2003. 22(3): p. 210-3.

[80] Chigbu, D.I., The management of allergic eye diseases in primary eye care. *Cont Lens Anterior Eye,* 2009. 32(6): p. 260-72.

[81] Moote, W. and H. Kim, Allergen-specific immunotherapy. *Allergy Asthma Clin Immunol,* 2011. 7 Suppl 1: p. S5.

[82] Broide, D.H., Immunomodulation of allergic disease. *Annu Rev Med,* 2009. 60: p. 279-91.

[83] Gentile, D. and D.P. Skoner, Sublingual immunotherapy in patients with allergic rhinoconjunctivitis. *Curr Allergy Asthma Rep,* 2011. 11(2): p. 131-8.

[84] Kasetsuwan, N., P. Chatchatee, and U. Reinprayoon, Efficacy of local conjunctival immunotherapy in allergic conjunctivitis. *Asian Pac J Allergy Immunol,* 2010. 28(4): p. 237-41.

[85] Morris, A.E. and G.D. Marshall, Jr., Safety of allergen immunotherapy: a review of premedication and dose adjustment. *Immunotherapy,* 2012. 4(3): p. 315-22.

[86] Collum, L.M., Vernal keratoconjunctivitis. *Acta Ophthalmol Scand Suppl,* 1999(228): p. 14-6.

Chapter 6

Allergic Conjunctivitis

Allergic conjunctivitis is caused by an allergen-induced inflammatory response in which allergens, such as pollens, ragweed, house dust mite, mold and animal dander interact with IgE bound to sensitized conjunctival mast cells resulting in mediator release and clinical manifestations of allergic conjunctivitis [1-3]. Allergic conjunctivitis affects more than 20% of the population [4]. The most common ocular allergies worldwide are seasonal allergic conjunctivitis (SAC) and perennial allergic conjunctivitis (PAC), with SAC being the most frequent form [5]. SAC is an intermittent IgE-mediated-condition and PAC is a persistent IgE-mediated condition of the conjunctiva [6]. Allergic conjunctivitis can have a profound effect on the quality of life and wellbeing of an individual. It affects learning performance in school-aged individuals and work productivity in adults [5, 7]. Allergic conjunctivitis is a bilateral, self-limiting conjunctival inflammatory process that occurs in sensitized individuals of either sex. Individuals with allergic conjunctivitis usually have a personal or family history of atopic disease, such as allergic rhinitis [5].

Pathomechanism

The pathogenesis of allergic conjunctivitis is predominantly an IgE-mediated hypersensitivity reaction. This occurs in three stages. The initial stage is referred to as the sensitization phase. The sensitization phase involves the initial exposure of the ocular surface to the allergens. The healthy conjunctiva epithelium acts as an impermeable barrier to the passage of allergens [8]. In order to initiate an allergic response, allergens need to cross the ocular surface to gain access to the conjunctival stromal [9]. It is of note that house dust mites, mold, and pollen allergens have protease activity. As such, the allergen source-derived proteases promote allergenicity [10]. Allergens such as house dust mite fecal pellets and pollen secrete serine proteases that activate protease-activated receptor-2 (PAR-2) in the conjunctival epithelium, an important regulator of conjunctival epithelial barrier permeability [8, 9]. PAR-2 upregulation dysregulates the epithelial barrier function, which results in increased permeability of the epithelium to the allergens. Thus, the allergens gain access into the subepithelial tissue where it is taken up by APCs [8, 11-13]. The biochemical processes initiated by the interaction between the antigen presenting cells and allergen, results in the development of allergen-specific IgE that becomes specific for that particular allergen. The IgE binds to the high affinity IgE receptors (FcεRI) located on the surface of mast cells and basophils. This primes the mast cells for response upon subsequent allergen exposure, completing the process of sensitization. The early phase response (EPR) of allergic conjunctivitis is an IgE-mediated reaction triggered by re-exposure to the same allergen that induced the sensitization of the mast cells. This involves allergen–induced cross-linking of allergen-specific IgE bound to the FcεRI on the sensitized mast cells. This triggers a biological cascade that causes changes in membrane calcium transport, and leads to disruption of the cell membrane and mast cell activation. The activated mast cell undergoes degranulation with release of mediators, such as histamine [14]. Furthermore, mast cell activation results in release of tryptase to promote further upregulation of PAR-2 [9]. Histamine release following mast cell degranulation is responsible for the signs and symptoms of allergic conjunctivitis [15]. The activation of histamine receptor on nerve endings by histamine induces pruritus while binding of histamine to histamine receptor on the vascular endothelium induces vasodilation (hyperemia) and increased vasopermeability (chemosis) [16]. IgE and mast cells play a major role in the disease mechanism of SAC and PAC [6, 7].

The histopathological and laboratory findings in allergic conjunctivitis revealed increased levels of mast cells in the conjunctival and increased levels of allergen-specific IgE and histamine [17, 18]. The tear level of eosinophil cationic protein (ECP), a specific marker of eosinophil activation, has been demonstrated to be elevated in SAC and PAC [19].

Clinical Presentation

The hallmark signs and symptoms of allergic conjunctivitis include itching, conjunctiva hyperemia, chemosis, mucoid or watery discharge, burning, redness, fine papillary hypertrophy, and eyelid swelling (Figures 1 and 2). The most bothersome symptom of allergic conjunctivitis is ocular itching and the most bothersome sign is redness [3, 20].

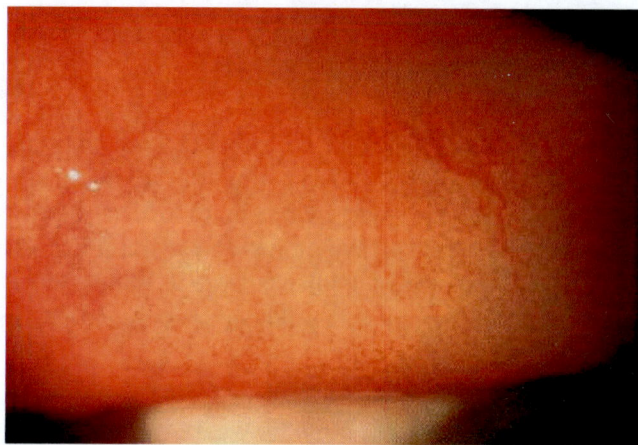

Figure 1. Fine papillary reaction in Allergic Conjunctivitis.

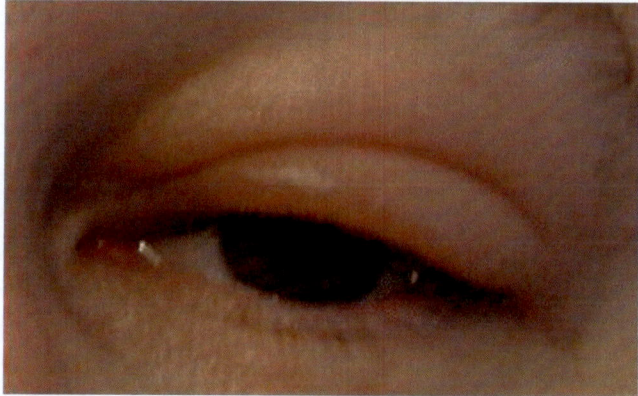

Figure 2. Eyelid Edema in Allergic Conjunctivitis (Photograph courtesy of Andrew S. Gurwood, O.D.).

Diagnosis

The diagnosis of allergic conjunctivitis is based on the constellation of clinical signs and symptoms. The skin prick testing or radioallergosorbent (RAST) test is a useful test for confirming the diagnosis of atopy [5]. Consulting with an allergist to assist in identifying the causative agents may be beneficial.

Management

The first line of therapy for patients with allergic conjunctivitis is to avoid the offending allergens. The primary aim of a non-pharmacological management approach (the first-line treatment of ocular allergy) to ocular allergy is to prevent the onset of symptoms and to minimize the effect of allergens. It includes avoidance of known allergens; saline irrigation; avoid eye rubbing; and palliative therapy with cold compresses and preservative-free ocular lubricants.

Patients should be advised to stay indoors and keep the windows closed or wear a filter mask if it is necessary for them to stay outside on days when the pollen count is high. They should also be advised to be more aware of the pollen count through the weather forecast; avoid cutting grass on windy days and when the pollen count is high; and avoid going near freshly cut grass during the height of the allergy season. Furthermore, the patient should be advised to avoid damp areas as these are potential breeding grounds for molds. They should be mindful to keep pets out of the bedroom, since their hair/fur can collect allergens and keep the kitchen and bathroom clean and dry, so as to minimize the growth and/or breeding of mold [21].

When avoidance fails, the clinician should recommend supportive and therapeutic anti-allergic therapy. It is good clinical practice to advise patients to use supportive therapies such as cool compresses, face washing and ocular lubricants as an adjunct to pharmacologic management. The clinician could advise the patient to keep preservative-free ocular lubricants in the refrigerator. The cold temperature of the refrigerated preservative-free ocular lubricants in conjunction with cool compresses induces vasoconstriction that counteracts the allergen-induced vasodilatation effect that causes chemosis and eyelid swelling. Additionally, preservative-free ocular lubricants dilute and flush away allergens, histamine and other inflammatory mediators that may encounter the ocular surface without having any impact on the activity of inflammatory mediators. They also form a barrier to inhibit allergen contact with the ocular surface [5, 22].

Therapeutic agents used for treating allergic conjunctivitis include antihistamines, topical NSAIDs, topical corticosteroids, topical mast cell stabilizers and topical antihistamine/ mast cell stabilizer combinations. Prescription and over-the-counter oral antihistamine can also play a role in reducing the overall allergic sensitivity of the body.

Mild to moderate cases of allergic conjunctivitis will respond to antihistamine, topical multimodal anti-allergic agents, topical mast cell stabilizers and supportive therapies. Individuals that present with hyperacute expressions of allergic conjunctivitis, severe allergic conjunctivitis or allergic conjunctivitis that is refractory to conventional anti-allergic therapy would benefit from short term topical steroidal therapy [23]. The pulse topical steroidal therapy can be tapered and discontinued, once the allergic inflammatory response is contained. However, it would be necessary to recommend the use of mast cell stabilizers or antihistamine/mast cell stabilizer combination agent for long-term management.

Patients who present with allergic rhinoconjunctivitis may benefit from using a nasal spray (e.g. azelastine hydrochloride nasal spray) or oral antihistamine (e.g. Claritin or Zyrtec) to provide therapeutic relief for the rhinitis and a topical multimodal anti-allergic ophthalmic agent to treat the allergic conjunctivitis [24, 25]. The clinical features of rhino-conjunctivitis are nasal itching, sneezing, rhinorrhea and congestion. The ocular allergic component of rhinoconjunctivitis includes itching, chemosis, redness, tearing and lid swelling. A clinical study demonstrated the superiority of antiallergic ophthalmic medication over antiallergic nasal spray in treating allergic conjunctivitis [16].

If the clinician decides to recommend systemic antihistamines, they may advise the patient to use preservative-free ocular lubricants in view of the fact that systemic antihistamines can reduce the aqueous component of the pre-ocular tear film. Systemic antihistamines have a long duration of action but have a delayed onset of action [7]. This is the reason clinicians are advised to treat allergic conjunctivitis with a topical anti-allergic ophthalmic agent.

Antihistamines, mast cell stabilizers and multiple action anti-allergic agents are sufficient to control the clinical manifestations of allergic conjunctivitis. However, pulse steroidal therapy will become necessary in severe or hyperacute cases. The major advantage of using topical multiple action anti-allergic ophthalmic agents is that the antihistamine will provide immediate therapeutic effect aimed at resolving the effects of the released histamine, while the mast cell stabilizer provides long term prophylaxis. Mast cell stabilizers are not effective in treating acute allergic conjunctivitis; however, they are beneficial when used prior to the expected exposure to allergen or allergy season since they require a loading period of weeks before antigen exposure for maximal efficacy [7]. Additionally, if the allergic conjunctivitis is not well controlled with conventional therapeutic modalities, allergen-specific immunotherapy could be beneficial for these patients who have evidence of specific IgE antibodies to clinically relevant allergens as demonstrated by skin prick or RAST test [26, 27].

Complications and Prognosis

Allergic conjunctivitis does not cause permanent ocular surface damage. It responds well to supportive and topical pharmacotherapy [5]. However, if left untreated, allergen induced disruption of the barrier function of the ocular surface epithelium can lead to increased permeability to allergens, which results in persistent activation of mast cells with eosinophil infiltration that leads to release of epitheliotoxic mediators [28]. Allergic conjunctivitis has a very favorable prognosis. However, the condition tends to reoccur.

References

[1] Sanchis-Merino, M., et al., Comparative efficacy of topical antihistamines in an animal model of early phase allergic conjunctivitis. *Exp Eye Res,* 2008. 86(5): p. 791-7.

[2] Scoper, S.V., et al., Perception and quality of life associated with the use of olopatadine 0.2% (Pataday) in patients with active allergic conjunctivitis. *Adv Ther,* 2007. 24(6): p. 1221-32.

[3] Leonardi, A., L. Motterle, and M. Bortolotti, Allergy and the eye. *Clin Exp Immunol,* 2008. 153 Suppl 1: p. 17-21.

[4] Aguilar, A., Comparative study of clinical efficacy and tolerance in seasonal allergic conjunctivitis management with 0.1% olopatadine hydrochloride versus 0.05% ketotifen fumarate. *Acta Ophthalmol Scand Suppl,* 2000(230): p. 52-5.

[5] Manzouri, B., et al., Pharmacotherapy of allergic eye disease. *Expert Opin Pharmacother,* 2006. 7(9): p. 1191-200.

[6] Leonardi, A., C. De Dominicis, and L. Motterle, Immunopathogenesis of ocular allergy: a schematic approach to different clinical entities. *Curr Opin Allergy Clin Immunol,* 2007. 7(5): p. 429-35.

[7] Pavesio, C. and H. Decory, Treatment of ocular inflammatory conditions with loteprednol etabonate. *Br J Ophthalmol,* 2008. 92(4): p. 455-9.

[8] Irkec, M.T. and B. Bozkurt, Molecular immunology of allergic conjunctivitis. Curr Opin Allergy Clin Immunol, 2012. 12(5): p. 534-9.

[9] Yeoh, S., et al., Increased conjunctival expression of protease activated receptor 2 (PAR-2) in seasonal allergic conjunctivitis: a role for abnormal conjunctival epithelial permeability in disease pathogenesis? *Br J Ophthalmol,* 2011. 95(9): p. 1304-8.

[10] Matsumura, Y., Role of Allergen Source-Derived Proteases in Sensitization via Airway Epithelial Cells. *J Allergy* (Cairo), 2012. 2012: p. 903659.

[11] Takai, T. and S. Ikeda, Barrier dysfunction caused by environmental proteases in the pathogenesis of allergic diseases. *Allergol Int,* 2011. 60(1): p. 25-35.

[12] Murphy, K.P., Travers, P., Walport, M., Allergy and Allergic Diseases, in Janeway's Immunobiology. 2012, *Garland Science:* New York. p. 571-610.

[13] Ohbayashi, M., et al., The Role of Histamine in Ocular Allergy. *Adv Exp Med Biol,* 2010. 709: p. 43-52.

[14] Abelson, M. and J. Greiner, Comparative efficacy of olopatadine 0.1% ophthalmic solution versus levocabastine 0.05% ophthalmic suspension using the conjunctival allergen challenge model. *Curr Med Res Opin,* 2004. 20(12): p. 1953-8.

[15] Abelson, M., L. Smith, and M. Chapin, Ocular allergic disease: mechanisms, disease sub-types, treatment. *Ocul Surf,* 2003. 1(3): p. 127-49.

[16] Rosenwasser, L., et al., A comparison of olopatadine 0.2% ophthalmic solution versus fluticasone furoate nasal spray for the treatment of allergic conjunctivitis. *Allergy Asthma Proc.* 29(6): p. 644-53.

[17] Reiss, J., et al., Allergic conjunctivitis. In: Pepose JS, Holland GN, Wilhelmus KR, editors. *Ocular infection and immunity.* 1996, St. Louis: Mosby. 345–58.

[18] Stahl, J., et al., Pathophysiology of ocular allergy: the roles of conjunctival mast cells and epithelial cells. *Curr Allergy Asthma Rep,* 2002. 2(4): p. 332-9.

[19] Jedrzejczak-Czechowicz, M., et al., Mast cell and eosinophil activation during early phase of grass pollen-induced ocular allergic reaction. *Allergy Asthma Proc,* 2011. 32(1): p. 43-8.

[20] Mah, F., et al., Efficacy and comfort of olopatadine 0.2% versus epinastine 0.05% ophthalmic solution for treating itching and redness induced by conjunctival allergen challenge. *Curr Med Res Opin,* 2007. 23(6): p. 1445-52.

[21] Kirkner, R., Lose the CAT...and Other Pearls from Allergists. *Review of Optometry,* 2001. 138(3): p. 94 - 98.

[22] Chigbu, D.I., The management of allergic eye diseases in primary eye care. *Contact Lens Anterior Eye,* 2009. 32(6): p. 260-72.

[23] Butrus, S. and R. Portela, Ocular allergy: diagnosis and treatment. *Ophthalmol Clin North Am,* 2005. 18(4): p. 485-92, v.

[24] Leonardi, A., Emerging drugs for ocular allergy. *Expert Opin Emerg Drugs,* 2005. 10(3): p. 505-20.

[25] Crampton, H.J., A comparison of the relative clinical efficacy of a single dose of ketotifen fumarate 0.025% ophthalmic solution versus placebo in inhibiting the signs and symptoms of allergic rhinoconjunctivitis as induced by the conjunctival allergen challenge model. *Clin Ther,* 2002. 24(11): p. 1800-8.

[26] Broide, D.H., Immunomodulation of allergic disease. *Annu Rev Med,* 2009. 60: p. 279-91.

[27] Moote, W. and H. Kim, Allergen-specific immunotherapy. *Allergy Asthma Clin Immunol,* 2011. 7 Suppl 1: p. S5.

[28] Hom, M.M., A.L. Nguyen, and L. Bielory, Allergic conjunctivitis and dry eye syndrome. *Ann Allergy Asthma Immunol,* 2012. 108(3): p. 163-6.

Chapter 7

Vernal Keratoconjunctivitis

Vernal keratoconjunctivitis (VKC) is a recurrent, bilateral, chronic allergic inflammation of the ocular surface affecting mainly children and young adults with a predominance in males [1, 2]. VKC is characterized by persistent conjunctival inflammation with an over-expression of mast cells, eosinophils, basophils, neutrophils, macrophages and lymphocytes [3, 4]. The three forms of the disease include palpebral, limbal, and mixed vernal keratoconjunctivitis [1]. The classification of VKC is based on the main site of the papillary reaction [5]. The palpebral form is seen predominantly in Caucasians, whereas the limbal variety is the predominant form in non-Caucasians [6, 7].

Patients with the palpebral or tarsal form of VKC present with giant papillae (i.e. papillae >1mm) on the upper tarsal conjunctiva [8]. The tarsal form is characterized by irregular sized hypertrophic papillae that lead to cobblestone appearance on the upper tarsal plate [9]. Vernal plaques are common complications. The palpebral form is most frequent in the temperate regions and is usually associated with a personal history of atopic disease [10]. Patients with limbal VKC present with gelatinous limbal infiltration and papillary reaction of the upper tarsal conjunctiva (i.e. papillae <1mm) [8]. The purely or predominantly limbal form of VKC is more common in non-Caucasian patients. Visual loss from corneal complications is uncommon [10-12]. Mixed VKC has both giant papillae on the upper tarsal conjunctiva and gelatinous infiltration of the limbus [8].

VKC is bilateral in more than 96% of cases [13]. It generally affects pre-pubescent children and young adults from warm climates of the Mediterranean, Africa, Middle East, Asia, and Central and South America [2, 3, 7, 14]. The male preponderance can be attributed to a possible role hormonal factors play in the development of VKC [9, 11, 15]. However, it usually resolves after puberty, about 4 to 10 years after onset, but progression towards atopic keratoconjunctivitis (AKC) can be observed at an adult age [2, 7, 9]. Although it reoccurs in spring and summer, Bonini and associates [3, 13] reported that more than 60% of patients with VKC had recurrences in the winter. It has been reported that the longer patients suffer from VKC, there is a high probability of the seasonal presentation evolving into a perennial form of the disease [13]. Thus, depending on the climate and allergic disposition of the patient, it can be active throughout the year [7]. It is of note that the perennial form occurs more frequently in hot countries whereas the chronic seasonal patterns occur mostly in the temperate regions as atmospheric conditions promote flare-ups in the spring and summer [2]. It has been reported that VKC is strongly associated with atopy in temperate regions/climates with a less marked association with atopy in the tropical regions [10]. VKC can be characterized by two distinct groups 1) those patients that have a positive personal and family history of other allergic conditions and 2) those patients that have no personal or family history of other allergic disorders [7, 9]. Approximately 50% of patients with VKC have a family history of allergic disorders such as asthma and rhinitis [13]. These patients have a positive response on standard allergen tests, such as skin prick or radioallergosorbent test (RAST), confirming that VKC is not solely an IgE mediated disease [3, 9, 16]. The overexpression of the cells and mediators of ocular allergy suggest that VKC may be a phenotypic model of up-regulation of the cytokine gene cluster on chromosome 5q. The cytokine gene cluster, through its products, which include IL-3, 4, 5 and granulocyte/macrophage-colony-stimulating factor, regulate the prevalence of Th2-lymphocyte [11].

Pathomechanism

The immunopathogenesis of VKC is multifactorial [15]. Studies have indicated that VKC is predominantly a Th2-lymphocyte-mediated allergic inflammatory disease with an overexpression of Th2-derived cytokines, chemokines, adhesion molecules, eosinophils, growth factors, fibroblast, enzymes, mast cell, macrophages, dendritic cells bearing IgE in the ocular surface, as well as tissue remodeling [1, 9, 11]. The production of Th2-lymphocyte derived cytokines favor a local hyperproduction of IgE, recruitment and activation of eosinophils and differentiation and activation of mast cells [9, 15, 17]. It has been reported that climatic, environmental, hormonal, genetic, and neural factors may influence the pathogenesis of VKC [5, 17, 18]. Studies have reported the involvement of neural factors such as substance P and neural growth factor (NGF) in the pathogenesis of VKC. The overexpression of nerve growth factor receptors in the conjunctiva coupled with high serum levels of NGF suggest a possible neural influence in the pathogenesis of VKC [3]. There is an over expression of estrogen and progesterone receptors in the conjunctiva of VKC patients suggesting possible involvement of sex hormones in the pathogenesis of VKC [3, 17, 19]. These hormones may bind to conjunctival receptors and exert a proinflammatory effect through the recruitment of eosinophils to the conjunctival tissue [3]. Thus, the influx of inflammatory cells and mediators to the conjunctiva leads to the clinical manifestations seen in VKC [20].

Patients with VKC have increased expression of adhesion molecules [9]; Langerhans' cells with increased expression of co-stimulatory molecules that may contribute to developing the Th2-lymphocyte-mediated conjunctival inflammation [9]; increased expression of chemokines, such as CXCL8 (IL-8), eotaxin, and RANTES [9]; an imbalance between plasminogen activators and plasminogen activator inhibitor (PAI) [21]; increased tear levels of histamine secondary to histamine-metabolizing enzyme and deficiency of histaminases [9]; a conjunctiva infiltrated with activated inflammatory cells that release their toxic mediators such as eosinophil cationic protein, eosinophil major basic protein, eosinophil peroxidase, eosinophil neurotoxin, neutrophil derived myleperoxidase, and MMP-2 and -9, which are capable of causing corneal epithelial damage [15]; an imbalance between MMP and their natural tissue inhibitor of metalloproteinase (TIMP), which may also contribute to the pathogenesis of conjunctival inflammation, tissue remodeling and corneal changes [4]; elevated serum levels of soluble ICAM-1 and soluble IL-2 receptor [22]; an over expression of Th-2-derived cytokines in both the tears and ocular surface [23]; increased levels of TNF-α, IL-4 and IL-13 that induces expression of ICAM-1on corneal and conjunctival epithelial cells [22]; reduced M1 muscarinic receptor and irregular distribution of M2 and M3 muscarinic receptors in conjunctival epithelium, which may lead to the production of mucus with a low water content and an increased stickiness [24]; and elevated levels of substance P, a basic mediator of neurogenic inflammation, in tears and plasma [24].

The increased tear levels of histamine have been reported to be associated with a defect in activity of the histaminases. This increase could explain why nonspecific histamine release occurs despite the absence of stimulation and exacerbates the effects of chronic eye rubbing [9]. Abelson and associates demonstrated that a defect in histaminases activity in tears and serum may be responsible for the onset and maintenance of the allergic inflammation associated with VKC [25].

VKC is also characterized by remodeling of the conjunctival tissues. This occurs secondary to excess extracellular matrix (ECM) deposition, subepithelial fibrosis, chronic cellular infiltration and epithelial thickening [4]. Th2-lymphocyte-derived cytokines (IL-4 and IL-13), pro-inflammatory cytokines (TNF-α, IL-1α and IL-1β), eosinophils, macrophages, matrix metalloproteinase, and growth factors (VEGF, TGF-β, bFGF, and PDGF) play an important role in the pathogenesis of tissue remodeling of the ocular surface of patients with VKC. The growth factors are expressed by conjunctival resident cells (epithelial cells, fibroblasts, mast cells) and inflammatory cells (eosinophils and macrophages) [7, 26-28]. The matrix metalloproteinase (MMP-2 and MMP-9) are expressed by eosinophils, macrophages, conjunctival resident cells, corneal epithelial cells and corneal fibroblasts. Th2-lymphocyte derived cytokines, pro-inflammatory cytokines and growth factors are responsible for the development of fibroproliferative lesions of the conjunctiva in VKC. These lesions occur as a result of hyperplasia of the conjunctival fibroblast, increased deposition of ECM molecules, and infiltration of inflammatory cells [7, 27-29].

Vascular endothelial growth factor (VEGF) plays a vital role in the process of angiogenesis and increases vascular permeability. Epithelial cells and inflammatory cells including eosinophils, monocytes and macrophages are the major cellular sources of VEGF. In the presence of VEGF, plasma proteins can leak into the extravascular space leading to edema and profound alterations in the extracellular matrix. TGF-β is able to stimulate fibroblast proliferation and enhance the synthesis of VEGF from conjunctival fibroblasts [7, 30].

Tissue-remodeling reactions produce giant papillae formation, hyperplasia of the epithelium with numerous epithelial ingrowths, extensive deposition of extracellular matrix components, peripheral corneal fibrovascular proliferation and superficial corneal changes [7, 11, 30].

Clinical Presentation

The clinical features of VKC include itching, burning, tearing, blepharospasm, pseudoptosis due to heavy giant papillae on the upper tarsal conjunctiva or at the limbus, photophobia, mucus hyper-secretion resulting in mucous discharge, filamentous mucus discharge, eyelid edema, chemosis, perilimbal conjunctival pigmentation, pseudogerontoxon, neovascularization of the cornea, cicatrizing conjunctivitis, blepharitis, the presence of aggregates of epithelial cells and eosinophils at the limbus (Horner-Trantas dots) and superficial keratitis [11, 14, 31, 32]. Bonini and colleagues [33] proposed a clinical grading to help physicians in the diagnosis and management of VKC. The **clinical manifestations of the mild form of VKC** includes occasional pruritus, mild tearing, mild discomfort including burning, mucoid discharge, mild photophobia, mild to moderate papillary reaction, mild corneal epithelial defects, subepithelial fibrosis of the conjunctiva and mild redness and edema of the eyelid. The **clinical manifestations of the moderate form of VKC** includes persistent itching, intermittent tearing, moderate discomfort, moderate mucoid discharge with the presence of crust upon awakening, moderate photophobia, moderate tarsal papillary hypertrophy and hyperemia with hazy view of the deep vessels, Horner-Trantas dots, moderate corneal epithelial defects with corneal neovascularization, moderate subepithelial fibrosis and moderate eyelid inflammation with meibomian gland dysfunction. The **clinical manifestations of the severe form of VKC** includes constant itching and tearing, severe discomfort, marked mucoid discharge with agglutination of the eyelids upon awakening, extreme photophobia, severe tarsal papillary hypertrophy and hyperemia obscuring the visualization of the deep tarsal vessels, severe corneal epithelial defects in the form of cornea erosion or ulceration with corneal neovascularization, numerous Horner-Trantas dots, the presence of symblepharon and severe inflammation of the eyelid [14, 33].

A **circumcorneal or perilimbal pigment** described as fine, golden brown pigmented limbal thickening is usually seen in VKC patients (figure 1). The color varies from faint to dark brown and is most frequently found in the area of the bulbar conjunctiva around the limbus but not in the tarsal conjunctiva. It is of note that there is an abundance of melanocytes in the limbus. Luk and associates suggested that the perilimbal conjunctival pigmentation observed in VKC patients may be due to growth factors or cytokines stimulating the melanocytes to produce the perilimbal pigment [34]. Thus, the perilimbal conjunctival hyperpigmentation could be due to proliferation of the melanocytes.

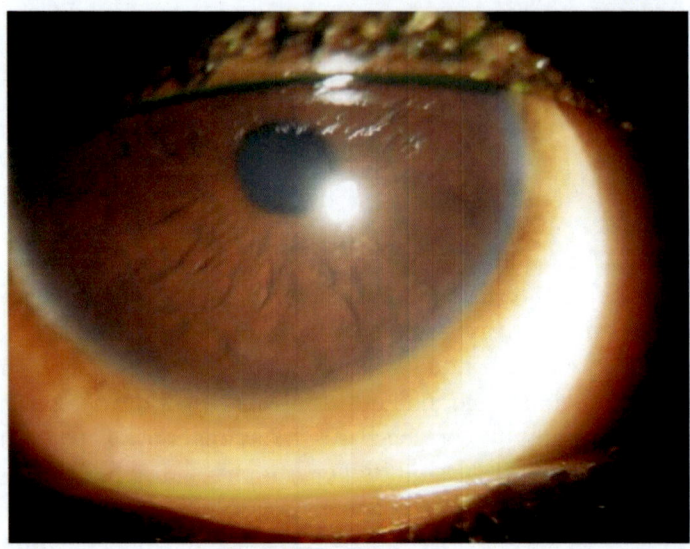

Figure 1. Perilimbal conjunctival pigmentation.

Conjunctival giant papillae in the superior tarsus and /or limbus are considered the hallmark of the disease (Figure 2) [5]. The papillae consists of conjunctival epithelium containing goblet cells, lymphocytes, plasma cells, eosinophils, mast cells, neutrophils, and newly formed vessels among excess fibrosis [35]. It has been reported that inflammation of the conjunctiva rather than mechanical factors plays a greater role in formation of giant papillae and exacerbation of VKC. Tissue remodeling is believed to be an important mechanism in giant papillary formation in VKC [36]. The conjunctival resident cells (epithelium and fibroblasts) are involved in the pathomechanisms leading to conjunctival giant papillae formation in VKC [15]. It is of note that there is an increase in type IV and type VII collagen in patients with VKC, which suggest that the tissue remodeling in VKC also involves the basement membrane [29]. The limbal form of the disease is characterized by multiple gelatinous yellow-gray limbal infiltrates (Figure 3). Limbal involvement in VKC includes limbal thickening or opacification, as well as the presence of limbal papillae, Horner-Trantas' dots and pannus of the superior limbus [9]. Horner-Trantas dots are usually found on the superior limbus in patients with limbal VKC. They are composed of clumps of necrotic eosinophils, neutrophils, and epithelial cells [37, 38]. The Horner-Trantas dots tend to appear when VKC is active and disappear when symptoms subside (figure 4) [39].

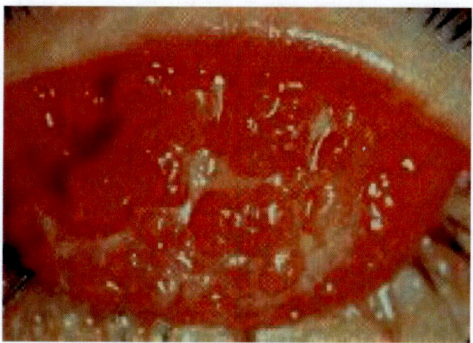

Figure 2. Giant papillae in Palpebral VKC (Photograph courtesy of Jeffrey S. Nyman, O.D.).

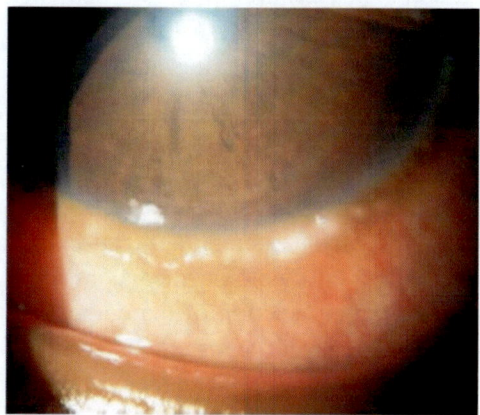

Figure 3. Gelatinous Limbal Infiltration in Limbal VKC.

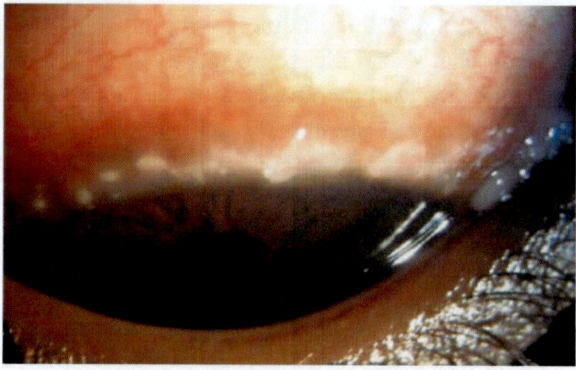

Figure 4. Gelatinous limbal infiltration and Horner-Trantas dots.

Corneal involvement occurs in more than 50% of patients with VKC. Although the cornea is an immunological privileged tissue, it contains antigen presenting cells such as macrophages and dendritic cells. The macrophages are located in the posterior corneal stroma. They express MHC class II-negative markers, as well as CD80⁻ and CD86⁻ markers. The mature dendritic cells expressing costimulatory and MHC class II-positive markers are present in the peripheral cornea, whereas immature dendritic cells expressing MHC class II-negative markers are present in the central cornea. Additionally, the cornea is composed of three structural cells (epithelial cells, fibroblasts, and endothelial cells) that may function as modulators of the allergic inflammation in VKC. It is of note that the cornea is not the primary site of allergic inflammation in VKC [27]. Th2-lymphocyte derived cytokines and pro-inflammatory cytokines stimulate the migration and proliferation of conjunctival and corneal fibroblasts. The activated corneal fibroblasts express eotaxin and vascular cell adhesion molecule (VCAM) -1 that mediate the infiltration and activation of eosinophil. The activated eosinophil releases MMP-2, MMP-9 and eosinophil-derived cytotoxic mediators. The active forms of MMP-2 and MMP-9 in tear film of VKC patients may play an important role in the pathogenesis of corneal lesions by mediating the degradation of collagen type IV and laminin of the corneal epithelial basement membrane. The exposure of the corneal epithelium to eosinophil-derived cytotoxic mediators and MMPs in the tear film can compromise the barrier function of the corneal epithelium, which in turn, leads to the development of persistent corneal epithelial defects in patients with VKC [7, 27, 28, 40]. The manifestations of corneal involvement in patients with VKC include punctate epithelial keratitis, epithelial macro-erosions, shield ulcer formation, plaque formation, corneal vascularization, secondary microbial keratitis, corneal ectasia, pseudogerontoxon and corneal opacification [8, 11, 41]. Punctate keratitis may be present in both limbal and palpebral forms but corneal shield ulcers are mostly seen in the tarsal form [9, 42]. In VKC, eosinophil-derived cytotoxic mediators and other inflammatory cells could damage the limbal stem cells, which in turn lead to recurrent corneal epithelial defects due to limbal stem cell dysfunction [43]. Corneal involvement in VKC with the development of ulceration can lead to sight-threatening complications, such as corneal scarring [37].

Shield ulcer is an oval or pentagonal shaped, superficial lesion located in the superior third of the cornea [8, 21]. A corneal shield ulcer is an uncommon but vision threatening complication that occurs in approximately 3%-11% of patients with VKC [3, 5, 11]. Corneal shield ulcer is usually common in patients with the tarsal form of VKC [5]. The pathogenesis of shield corneal ulcers is believed to involve a combination of chronic mechanical abrading of the corneal epithelium by giant papillae on the upper tarsal conjunctiva and epithelial toxicity from inflammatory mediators secreted by eosinophils and mast cells [8, 44, 45]. Additionally, activated corneal fibroblasts play a role in the development of shield ulcer, as it secretes MMP that degrades the collagen of the corneal stroma [46]. Eosinophil major basic protein (EMBP) is an inflammatory mediator that is capable of inhibiting corneal epithelial wound healing [8]. The deposition of EMBP on the denuded Bowman's layer leads to the development of a dense plaque [44], and as such, EMBP plays a role in the formation and persistence of VKC-related shield ulcers [47]. Punctate epithelial erosions that evolve into coarse epithelial keratopathy precede shield ulcers. Continued damage to the epithelium leads to the development of a frank corneal abrasion (macroerosion). An ulcer with a transparent base will form when the damage extends through the epithelium and basement membrane into the Bowman's layer. As the disease progresses, inflammatory debris is deposited on the base of the ulcer giving the ulcer a translucent appearance. The filling of the ulcer cavity with inflammatory debris eventually leads to the formation of an elevated plaque that extends above the level of the surrounding epithelium [8]. Cameron classified shield ulcers on the basis of their clinical characteristics, response to treatment and complications. Grade I corneal shield ulcers have a clear or transparent base. They have a favorable

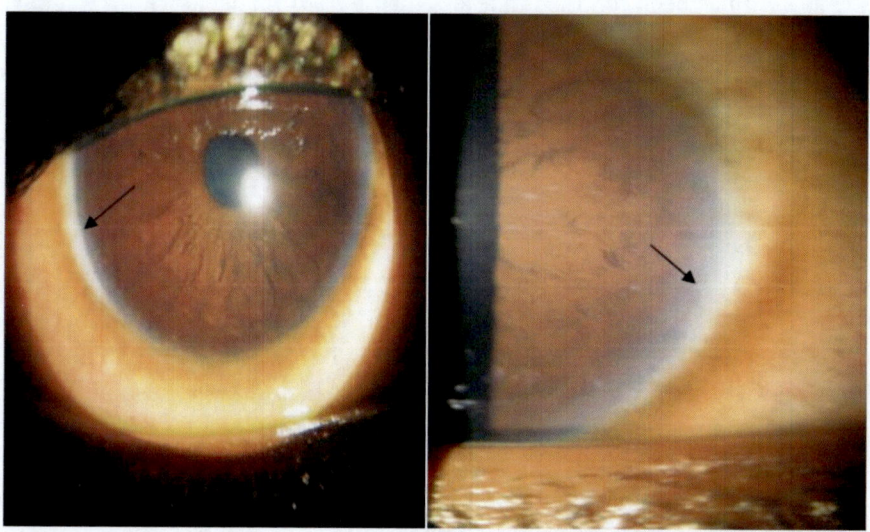

Figure 5. Pseudodgerotoxon.

outcome and re-epithelialize with only mild scarring. Grade II corneal shield ulcers have a translucent base with inflammatory debris at the base. They respond poorly to medical therapy and exhibit delayed re-epithelialization. Grade III corneal shield ulcers have elevated plaques. They are resistant to medical therapy and usually require surgical removal [8, 48, 49]. Corneal plaques occur due to the continuous deposition of mucus and inflammatory products on the shield ulcer [8].

Pseudogerontoxon is a localized grey-white lipid deposition in the anterior stroma of the peripheral cornea (figure 5). It resembles a small segment of arcus senilis. It results from prolonged limbal infiltration and altered limbal permeability secondary to limbal giant papillae [9, 11, 50]. It is seen in individuals with limbal vernal or atopic keratoconjunctivitis. It may be considered the only clinical evidence of previous allergic eye disease [50].

Diagnosis

The diagnosis of VKC is based on the constellation of clinical signs and symptoms. In difficult cases, tear or conjunctival cytology could be useful in assessing the type and number of cells involved in the conjunctival inflammation. Skin prick test or RAST are not considered useful in diagnosing VKC since it has been reported that less than 50% of patients with VKC have negative results on these tests [3, 15].

The differential diagnoses of VKC include seasonal allergic conjunctivitis (SAC), perennial allergic conjunctivitis (PAC), giant papillary conjunctivitis (GPC) and atopic keratoconjunctivitis (AKC). Unlike VKC, the pathogenesis of allergic conjunctivitis is predominantly an IgE-mediated hypersensitivity reaction; moreover, eosinophil and Th2-lymphocytes are unlikely to play a major role in the pathogenesis of allergic conjunctivitis, as noted by the absence of corneal damage in SAC and PAC [7, 51]. Although the histological appearance of the conjunctiva in VKC and GPC is almost identical, the main difference is that the number of eosinophils and basophils is greater in VKC than in GPC [7, 52, 53]. The level of EMBP, which may be responsible for injury to the corneal epithelium, is increased in patients with VKC but not in those with GPC [7, 52]. The perennial nature of the atopic keratoconjunctivitis distinguishes it from vernal keratoconjunctivitis, which typically has a seasonal pattern. Furthermore, AKC tends to have lower eyelid and inferior palpebral conjunctival involvement and begin in the late teens, whereas VKC is characterized by superior tarsal conjunctival papillary hypertrophy and tends to affect mostly children and young adult males [7, 54].

Management

The goal of therapy is to suppress the allergic inflammatory process. The primary form of therapy for patients with VKC is identification and avoidance of allergens. The avoidance of allergens or exposure to trigger factors such as sun, salt water, wind or dust with the use of sunglasses, hats, visors and swimming goggles may be beneficial. Frequent hand and face washing is also beneficial [9, 15].

The supportive therapy of VKC includes avoiding the trigger factors, avoiding eye rubbing, applying cool compress, saline irrigation to wash out allergens, and administering preservative-free ocular lubricants [55]. Chronic eye rubbing and activation of metalloproteinase may play a role in the development of keratoconus in VKC [9]. Therefore, it is important to counsel patients about avoiding eye rubbing [7]. Totan and colleagues [56] reported that approximately 27% of patients with VKC in their study had keratoconus, whereas Khan and colleagues [57] reported an incidence of 7%. The higher incidence reported by Totan et al. could be due to their use of computer-assisted videokeratographic maps that aided in the detection of subclinical keratoconus in patients with VKC, which could be overlooked using traditional methods such as biomicroscopy and keratoscope [56]. Therefore, evaluation of patients with VKC for subtle signs of keratoconus could be considered an important aspect of the management plan [7]. Preservative-free ocular lubricants aid in stabilization of the tear film, while diluting and/or flushing away allergens and allergic mediators [9]. Patients with a history of VKC should be started on prophylactic therapy with a multimodal anti-allergy pharmaceutical agent prior to the allergy season or should remain on the therapy all year round, depending on the allergic exposure and duration of the allergic expression. Educating patients and/or their parents about the disease process and the chronic, recurrent nature of VKC, as well as possible identification of trigger factors is an important aspect of management [11, 17]. An effective treatment and management plan will focus on preventing the degranulation of mast cells, as well as controlling or minimizing the effects of the mediators released by the mast cells.

Therapeutic measures are required to avoid the longstanding permanent inflammatory sequelae, fibrovascular reaction, new collagen deposition, tissue inflammation, tissue remodeling and permanent visual damage [2]. The chronicity and severity of the disease, warrants a combination of supportive and pharmacological treatment [9]. Standard pharmacologic treatment of VKC is based on the use of topical anti-allergic pharmaceutical agents and anti-inflammatory preparations [5]. Patients with mild VKC may benefit from supportive therapy as well as topical multimodal anti-allergic agents to provide symptomatic relief. However, a pulse topical steroidal therapy will become necessary to control the inflammation, if the anti-allergic therapy does not provide satisfactory therapeutic relief. Patients with moderate or severe VKC require concurrent use of topical steroids and multimodal anti-allergic agents to achieve an adequate therapeutic effect. Topical corticosteroids with a proven safety profile such as loteprednol etabonate has been shown to be effective in controlling the chronic allergic inflammatory process in VKC. The maximum strength topical corticosteroid, such as prednisolone acetate 1.0% ophthalmic suspension could be considered when the moderate strength topical steroids or soft topical steroids are not effective in controlling the allergic inflammation [58]. Treatment with systemic corticosteroids may become necessary when individuals present with severe VKC that does not respond to conventional topical therapy [3, 9].

Topical cyclosporine A has been proven to be effective in the long-term treatment of both limbal and tarsal VKC [9]. Although cyclosporine ophthalmic emulsion may be considered a suitable alternative to corticosteroids, in the presence of corneal complications caused by epithelial toxic mediators, such as EMBP, topical steroidal therapy is the preferred choice [3, 9, 15, 58, 59], since the therapeutic effect of dampening the inflammatory process is achieved more rapidly with steroidal therapy. It has been demonstrated that topical cyclosporine A 0.5%-2% used 4 times a day, may represent an alternative to steroidal therapy in severe forms of VKC [3]. Keklikci and associates noted that administration of topical cyclosporine A 0.05% for 3 months was remarkably effective at improving signs and symptoms in VKC. A low concentration of topical cyclosporine was used with no systemic adverse effects recorded [14]. Spadavecchia and colleagues also demonstrated the efficacy of 1.25% and 1.0% topical cyclosporine in the treatment of severe VKC with successful outcome. In their study, none of the patients had any major side effects or need for rescue topical steroidal therapy [18].

Patients with shield ulcer or corneal epithelial compromise secondary to VKC would benefit from using a therapeutic bandage contact lens as an adjunctive therapy. The objective of using a therapeutic bandage contact lens is to reduce the effect of the mechanical chafing between the papillae on the superior tarsal conjunctiva and corneal epithelial surface. Additionally, therapeutic bandage contact lens relieves pain, promotes corneal epithelial healing and protects the fragile corneal epithelium during the healing process [60]. The clinician could prescribe prophylactic antibiotics and recommend preservative-free ocular lubricants as essential adjunctive therapeutic strategies when therapeutic bandage contact lenses are used [61]. The complications of therapeutic bandage contact lens use include infection, hypoxia, hypercapnia, tissue necrosis in the cornea, microcyst formation, decreased corneal sensation and pannus formation [60]. The management strategies of shield ulcers are often guided by the severity of the lesion. Grade I shield ulcer respond to pharmaceutical therapy consisting of topical steroid, antibiotic prophylactics and mast cell stabilizers with concurrent use of a bandage contact lens to promote re-epithelialization. Grade II shield ulcers with translucent or opaque bases require medical therapy to control the active VKC and surgical intervention to remove the inflammatory material at the base of the ulcer [8]. Grade III lesions with elevated plaque above the level of the surrounding epithelium usually respond well to surgical therapy [8]. A combination of pharmaceutical and/or surgical intervention is required to achieve re-epithelialization in these cases. The rationale for surgical intervention is to remove the inflammatory material at the base and margins of the vernal corneal ulcer, as it mechanically prevents re-epithelialization as well as act as a toxin to the epithelium. This inflammatory material has been shown to be composed of eosinophil-derived cytotoxic mediators whose cytotoxic properties hinder wound healing [8, 48].

Complications and Prognosis

Visual loss may be due to corneal neovascularization, central corneal scars, irregular astigmatism, keratoconus, and steroid-induced cataract and glaucoma [15, 20]. Amblyopia seen among VKC patients may be caused by corneal opacity or refractive changes producing corneal curvature alterations or the development of keratoconus [11]. Although limbal infiltrates may cause transitory modifications of corneal astigmatism, keratoconus is the most frequent corneal ectasia associated with VKC.

Delays in treatment as well as under-treatment in moderate and severe cases of VKC may lead to the development of significant morbidity. Prompt diagnosis and appropriate treatment may prevent the development of permanent ocular complications and visual loss [21, 59].

The long-term prognosis of patients with VKC is generally good. However, 6% of patients develop visual impairment secondary to corneal damage, steroid-induced cataract and glaucoma, microbial keratitis or limbal tissue hyperplasia [2, 11, 13]. Patients with shield ulcers without plaque formation usually undergo rapid re-epithelialization, resulting in an excellent visual outcome, whereas patients with shield ulcers with plaque formation have a poor visual prognosis [8, 41]. It has been reported that the bulbar form of VKC is said to have a worse long-term prognosis than the tarsal form [3, 13, 17]. However, the majority of patients with VKC have spontaneous resolution of the disease after puberty without any further symptoms or visual complication [3].

References

[1]   Abu El-Asrar, A.M., et al., Gelatinase B in vernal keratoconjunctivitis. *Arch Ophthalmol,* 2001. 119(10): p. 1505-11.

[2]   Bremond-Gignac, D., et al., Prevalence of vernal keratoconjunctivitis: a rare disease? *Br J Ophthalmol,* 2008. 92(8): p. 1097-102.

[3]   Bonini, S., et al., Vernal keratoconjunctivitis. *Eye,* 2004. 18(4): p. 345-51.

[4]   Leonardi, A., et al., Matrix metalloproteases in vernal keratoconjunctivitis, nasal polyps and allergic asthma. *Clin Exp Allergy,* 2007. 37(6): p. 872-9.

[5]   Lambiase, A., et al., Prospective, multicenter demographic and epidemiological study on vernal keratoconjunctivitis: a glimpse of ocular surface in Italian population. *Ophthalmic Epidemiol,* 2009. 16(1): p. 38-41.

[6]   Coutu, R.B., Treatment of vernal keratoconjunctivitis: a retrospective clinical case study. Wallace F. Molinari Ocular Pharmacology Award. *Optom Vis Sci,* 1991. 68(7): p. 561-4.

[7]   Chigbu, D.I. and S. Sandrasekaramudaly-Brown, Ocular surface disease: a case of vernal keratoconjunctivitis. *Cont Lens Anterior Eye,* 2011. 34(1): p. 39-44.

[8]   Cameron, J.A., Shield ulcers and plaques of the cornea in vernal keratoconjunctivitis. *Ophthalmology,* 1995. 102(6): p. 985-93.

[9] Leonardi, A. and A.G. Secchi, Vernal keratoconjunctivitis. *Int Ophthalmol Clin,* 2003. 43(1): p. 41-58.

[10] Tuft, S.J., et al., Limbal vernal keratoconjunctivitis in the tropics. *Ophthalmology,* 1998. 105(8): p. 1489-93.

[11] Kumar, S., Vernal keratoconjunctivitis: a major review. *Acta Ophthalmol,* 2009. 87(2): p. 133-47.

[12] Holsclaw, D.S., et al., Supratarsal injection of corticosteroid in the treatment of refractory vernal keratoconjunctivitis. *Am J Ophthalmol,* 1996. 121(3): p. 243-9.

[13] Bonini, S., et al., Vernal keratoconjunctivitis revisited: a case series of 195 patients with long-term followup. *Ophthalmology,* 2000. 107(6): p. 1157-63.

[14] Keklikci, U., et al., Efficacy of topical cyclosporin A 0.05% in conjunctival impression cytology specimens and clinical findings of severe vernal keratoconjunctivitis in children. *Jpn J Ophthalmol,* 2008. 52(5): p. 357-62.

[15] Bonini, S., A. Lambiase, and R. Sgrulletta, Allergic chronic inflammation of the ocular surface in vernal keratoconjunctivitis. *Curr Opin Allergy Clin Immunol,* 2003. 3(5): p. 381-7.

[16] Iovieno, A., et al., Preliminary evidence of the efficacy of probiotic eye-drop treatment in patients with vernal keratoconjunctivitis. *Graefes Arch Clin Exp Ophthalmol,* 2008. 246(3): p. 435-41.

[17] Akinsola, F.B., et al., Vernal keratoconjunctivitis at Guinness Eye Centre, Luth (a five year study). *Nig Q J Hosp Med,* 2008. 18(1): p. 1-4.

[18] Spadavecchia, L., et al., Efficacy of 1.25% and 1% topical cyclosporine in the treatment of severe vernal keratoconjunctivitis in childhood. *Pediatr Allergy Immunol, 2006.* 17(7): p. 527-32.

[19] Bonini, S., et al., Estrogen and progesterone receptors in vernal keratoconjunctivitis. *Ophthalmology,* 1995. 102(9): p. 1374-9.

[20] Gupta, A., A. Sharma, and K. Mohan, Mycotic keratitis in non-steroid exposed vernal keratoconjunctivitis. *Acta Ophthalmol Scand,* 1999. 77(2): p. 229-31.

[21] Gedik, S., Y.A. Akova, and S. Gur, Secondary bacterial keratitis associated with shield ulcer caused by vernal conjunctivitis. *Cornea,* 2006. 25(8): p. 974-6.

[22] Irkeç, M. and B. Bozkurt, Epithelial cells in ocular allergy. *Curr Allergy Asthma Rep,* 2003. 3(4): p. 352-7.

[23] Leonardi, A., et al., Urokinase plasminogen activator, uPa receptor, and its inhibitor in vernal keratoconjunctivitis. *Invest Ophthalmol Vis Sci,* 2005. 46(4): p. 1364-70.

[24] Motterle, L., et al., Altered expression of neurotransmitter receptors and neuromediators in vernal keratoconjunctivitis. *Arch Ophthalmol,* 2006. 124(4): p. 462-8.

[25] Abelson, M.B., et al., Histaminase activity in patients with vernal keratoconjunctivitis. *Ophthalmology,* 1995. 102(12): p. 1958-63.

[26] Leonardi, A., et al., Growth factors and collagen distribution in vernal keratoconjunctivitis. *Invest Ophthalmol Vis Sci,* 2000. 41(13): p. 4175-81.

[27] Fukuda, K., et al., Fibroblasts as local immune modulators in ocular allergic disease. *Allergol Int,* 2006. 55(2): p. 121-9.

[28] Kumagai, N., et al., Role of structural cells of the cornea and conjunctiva in the pathogenesis of vernal keratoconjunctivitis. *Prog Retin Eye Res,* 2006. 25(2): p. 165-87.

[29] Solomon, A., I. Puxeddu, and F. Levi-Schaffer, Fibrosis in ocular allergic inflammation: recent concepts in the pathogenesis of ocular allergy. *Curr Opin Allergy Clin Immunol,* 2003. 3(5): p. 389-93.

[30] Abu El-Asrar, A.M., et al., Immunopathogenesis of conjunctival remodelling in vernal keratoconjunctivitis. *Eye,* 2006. 20(1): p. 71-9.

[31] Corum, I., et al., Efficiency of olopatadine hydrochloride 0.1% in the treatment of vernal keratoconjunctivitis and goblet cell density. *J Ocul Pharmacol Ther,* 2005. 21(5): p. 400-5.

[32] Rao, S.K., et al., Perilimbal bulbar conjunctival pigmentation in vernal conjunctivitis: prospective evaluation of a new clinical sign in an Indian population. *Cornea,* 2004. 23(4): p. 356-9.

[33] Bonini, S., et al., Clinical grading of vernal keratoconjunctivitis. *Curr Opin Allergy Clin Immunol,* 2007. 7(5): p. 436-41.

[34] Luk, F.O., et al., Perilimbal conjunctival pigmentation in Chinese patients with vernal keratoconjunctivitis. *Eye,* 2008. 22(8): p. 1011-4.

[35] Asano-Kato, N., et al., TGF-beta1, IL-1beta, and Th2 cytokines stimulate vascular endothelial growth factor production from conjunctival fibroblasts. *Exp Eye Res,* 2005. 80(4): p. 555-60.

[36] Kato, N., et al., Mechanisms of giant papillary formation in vernal keratoconjunctivitis. *Cornea,* 2006. 25(10 Suppl 1): p. S47-52.

[37] Ohbayashi, M., et al., The Role of Histamine in Ocular Allergy. *Adv Exp Med Biol,* 2010. 709: p. 43-52.

[38] Bielory, B. and L. Bielory, Atopic dermatitis and keratoconjunctivitis. *Immunol Allergy Clin North Am,* 2010. 30(3): p. 323-36.

[39] Friedlaender, M.H., Ocular allergy. *Curr Opin Allergy Clin Immunol,* 2011. 11(5): p. 477-82.

[40] Fukuda, K., et al., Inhibition of matrix metalloproteinase-3 synthesis in human conjunctival fibroblasts by interleukin-4 or interleukin-13. *Invest Ophthalmol Vis Sci,* 2006. 47(7): p. 2857-64.

[41] Kumar, S., Combined therapy for vernal shield ulcer. *Clin Exp Optom,* 2008. 91(1): p. 111-4.

[42] Cameron, J.A., A.A. Al-Rajhi, and I.A. Badr, Corneal ectasia in vernal keratoconjunctivitis. *Ophthalmology,* 1989. 96(11): p. 1615-23.

[43] Sangwan, V.S., et al., Vernal keratoconjunctivitis with limbal stem cell deficiency. *Cornea,* 2011. 30(5): p. 491-6.

[44] Solomon, A., et al., Surgical management of corneal plaques in vernal keratoconjunctivitis: a clinicopathologic study. *Cornea,* 2004. 23(6): p. 608-12.

[45] Cameron, J.A. and P.B. Mullaney, Amblyopia resulting from shield ulcers and plaques of the cornea in vernal keratoconjunctivitis. *J Pediatr Ophthalmol Strabismus,* 1997. 34(4): p. 261-2.

[46] Irkec, M.T. and B. Bozkurt, Molecular immunology of allergic conjunctivitis. *Curr Opin Allergy Clin Immunol,* 2012. 12(5): p. 534-9.

[47] Trocme, S.D., et al., Eosinophil granule major basic protein deposition in corneal ulcers associated with vernal keratoconjunctivitis. *Am J Ophthalmol,* 1993. 115(5): p. 640-3.

[48] Ozbek, Z., A.Z. Burakgazi, and C.J. Rapuano, Rapid healing of vernal shield ulcer after surgical debridement: A case report. *Cornea,* 2006. 25(4): p. 472-3.

[49] Pelegrin, L., et al., Superficial keratectomy and amniotic membrane patch in the treatment of corneal plaque of vernal keratoconjunctivitis. *Eur J Ophthalmol,* 2008. 18(1): p. 131-3.

[50] Jeng, B.H., J.P. Whitcher, and T.P. Margolis, Pseudogerontoxon. *Clin Experiment Ophthalmol,* 2004. 32(4): p. 433-4.

[51] Pavesio, C. and H. Decory, Treatment of ocular inflammatory conditions with loteprednol etabonate. *Br J Ophthalmol,* 2008. 92(4): p. 455-9.

[52] Allansmith, M.R. and R.N. Ross, Giant papillary conjunctivitis. *Int Ophthalmol Clin,* 1988. 28(4): p. 309-16.

[53] Donshik, P., Giant papillary conjunctivitis. *Trans Am Ophthalmol Soc,* 1994. 92: p. 687-744.

[54] Casey, R. and M.B. Abelson, Atopic keratoconjunctivitis. *Int Ophthalmol Clin,* 1997. 37(2): p. 111-7.

[55] Verin, P.H., I.D. Dicker, and B. Mortemousque, Nedocromil sodium eye drops are more effective than sodium cromoglycate eye drops for the long-term management of vernal keratoconjunctivitis. *Clin Exp Allergy,* 1999. 29(4): p. 529-36.

[56] Totan, Y., et al., Incidence of keratoconus in subjects with vernal keratoconjunctivitis: a videokeratographic study. *Ophthalmology,* 2001. 108(4): p. 824-7.

[57] Khan, M.D., et al., Incidence of keratoconus in spring catarrh. *Br J Ophthalmol,* 1988. 72(1): p. 41-3.

[58] Chigbu, D.I., The management of allergic eye diseases in primary eye care. *Cont Lens Anterior Eye,* 2009. 32(6): p. 260-72.

[59] Collum, L.M., Vernal keratoconjunctivitis. *Acta Ophthalmol Scand Suppl,* 1999(228): p. 14-6.

[60] Foulks, G.N., T. Harvey, and C.V. Raj, Therapeutic contact lenses: the role of high-Dk lenses. *Ophthalmol Clin North Am,* 2003. 16(3): p. 455-61.

[61] Lemp, M.A. and L. Bielory, Contact lenses and associated anterior segment disorders: dry eye disease, blepharitis, and allergy. *Immunol Allergy Clin North Am,* 2008. 28(1): p. 105-17, vi-vii.

Chapter 8

Atopic Keratoconjunctivitis

Atopic keratoconjunctivitis (AKC), a type I and type IV hypersensitivity reaction, is a bilateral chronic inflammatory disease of the ocular surface and eyelid. It is characterized by chronic conjunctivitis and progressive corneal infiltration with corneal neovascularization and fibrosis secondary to chronic epithelial disease and limbal stem cell dysfunction [1-4]. AKC, a sight-threatening ocular manifestation of a systemic altered immune response, is often associated with atopic dermatitis and with other allergic conditions [5-7]. It may persist for many years and has the potential to cause ocular surface complications with potentially blinding sequelae [2, 8]. AKC is the most severe and chronic form of allergy-related disorder of the ocular surface. Calonge and colleagues suggested that AKC is a chronic ocular surface inflammatory condition that atopic dermatitis patients may suffer at any point in the course of their dermatologic disease, independently of its degree of severity [9]. AKC is known to occur in 25% − 40% of patients with atopic dermatitis [4, 10]. Atopic dermatitis is a pruritic skin condition that affects 3% of the population worldwide [4]. The manifestations of AKC begin in the late teens or early twenties with a peak incidence between the ages of 30 and 50 years. It is more common in males. AKC has a perennial pattern of occurrence with exacerbations more common in the winter months [10, 11]. Patients with AKC have an inherited predisposition to atopy. There is a family history of allergic disorders such as asthma [10].

Pathomechanism

The pathogenesis of AKC is multifactorial. Genetic factors, antigen sensitization, neural factors, Th-lymphocytes, cytokines, hormonal factors and conjunctival hyper-reactivity all have an influence on the pathogenesis [7]. The immunopathophysiology of AKC involves chronic IgE-mediated mast cell degranulation and Th-lymphocyte-mediated immune mechanisms [10, 12, 13]. AKC is mediated by T-lymphocytes, eosinophils, mast cells, Th-lymphocyte derived cytokines and other inflammatory cells [14, 15]. In AKC, it has been shown that there is an over-expression of mucosal type mast cells and eosinophils in the conjunctiva [12].

Histopathological and laboratory findings of AKC revealed mast cells, eosinophils, elevated serum IgE, and Th-lymphocytes in the conjunctival epithelium [11, 16]; goblet cell proliferation [11, 16]; chronic mononuclear cell infiltration of the substantia propria [16]; elevated levels of TNF-α, IFN-γ, IL-2, IL-4, IL-5, and IL-10 in the tears [7, 11, 17]; significant levels of ECP, eosinophil neurotoxin and IL-2 receptors in the serum [7]; the presence of eotaxin and its receptor, CCR3, in the tears [7]; over-expression of IL-4, IL-8 and GM-CSF levels in conjunctival tissues [12]; upregulation of ocular surface ICAM-1 [1]; up-regulation of RANTES [1, 12]; increased degranulation of neutrophil and eosinophil resulting in release of toxic mediators that could damage the ocular surface [18]; high levels of IgE in tears and serum [13, 19]; and significant reduction in MUC5AC mRNA expression [20].

In AKC, the Th-lymphocytes are the primary mediators and effectors of tissue damage. There is recruitment of other cell types, including mast cells, eosinophils, and basophils which produce various allergic and inflammatory mediators. The chronically elevated levels of these cells and other mediators derived from them contribute significantly to the chronic damage seen in AKC [18, 21].

Patients with severe AKC showed marked staining for hexanoyl-lysine and 4-hydroxy-2-nonenal antibodies produced via lipid peroxidation in cells. Oxidative free radicals, produced by macrophages, neutrophils and eosinophils, can cause oxidative stress on the ocular surface, which in turn, induces lipid peroxidation that causes ocular surface inflammation [22].

Clinical Presentation

The most common complaints of patients with AKC are bilateral ocular itching, burning, and tearing. The symptoms are usually perennial [12]. The clinical features of AKC include papillary hypertrophy usually located on the lower tarsal conjunctiva; Dennie-Morgan lines involving the skin of the eyelid results in a single or double infraorbital crease secondary to edema; chemosis; limbal gelatinous hyperplasia; stringy discharge due to the accumulation of cellular debris, fibrin, and mucin; conjunctiva hyperemia; secondary staphylococcal blepharitis; and varying degrees of conjunctival and corneal involvement [4, 10, 11, 13]. It is of note that bilateral involvement with abundant mucoid discharge is the rule [11].

Calonge and colleagues [9] proposed a clinical grading to help physicians in the diagnosis and management of AKC. Patients with **milder forms of AKC (Grade I)** present with mild/or occasional itching, burning and photophobia. The clinical signs include anterior blepharitis, hyperemia/edema/papillae of the tarsal conjunctiva and superficial punctate keratitis. Patients with **mild-to-moderate forms of AKC (Grade II)** present with mildly persistent or moderate itching, burning and photophobia. In addition to grade I signs, these patients present with meibomian gland dysfunction, hyperemia/edema in the bulbar-limbal conjunctiva region (ciliary injection) and non-persistent corneal epithelial defects. Patients with **moderate forms of AKC (Grade III)** present with moderately persistent itching, burning and photophobia. In addition to the grade II signs, patients with grade III disease present with meibomianitis, conjunctival subepithelial fibrosis, and neovascularization, scarring and thinning of the cornea. Persistent corneal epithelial defects are also present. Patients with **severe forms of AKC (Grade IV)** present with severe itching, burning and photophobia. In addition to the grade III signs, these individuals present with conjunctival cicatrizing changes such as fornix foreshortening or symblepharon [9].

AKC is a chronic disease associated with alterations in the mucin layer of the tear film. This causes increased mucus discharge, corneal epithelial disease and ocular surface desiccation [7]. Ocular surface mucins are believed to provide a barrier to prevent pathogens and particulate matter from entering the ocular surface epithelium. Mucin may play an important role in increasing the tear film stability and the hydration of the ocular surface [20]. It has been shown that conjunctival squamous metaplasia, tear film instability and goblet cell loss in AKC are associated with a decrease in mucin 5AC and upregulation of mucin 1, 2 and 4 gene expressions. This may explain the lower stability and wettability of the tear film observed in AKC patients [7, 20].

Squamous metaplasia is a pathologic trans-differentiation of nonkeratinized-stratified epithelium into a nonsecretory, keratinized epithelium [23]. Additionally, IL-1β and IFN-γ play a pathogenic role in T-lymphocyte mediated squamous metaplasia [24].

The eyelid and periorbital manifestations in AKC include eczema of the periorbital skin and cheeks; hyperpigmentation of the periocular skin; atopic-related eyelid dermatitis and blepharitis; meibomianitis; eyelid margin keratinization; trichiasis/distichiasis; madarosis; rosacea-related blepharitis; ectropion; entropion; profound eyelid edema with Dennie-Morgan folds; upper eyelid ptosis; fissures in the lateral canthus due to excessive eyelid rubbing; and staphylococcal blepharitis [3, 10, 25]. Staphylococcus aureus colonization is common in AKC [7]. Lipases originating from bacteria colonizing the lid margin are believed to degrade some of the lipids as they are secreted, altering the composition of the tear film lipids [17]. Additionally, S. aureus can induce Th2-lymphocyte type immune responses by upregulating and activating TLR2. Thus, S. aureus colonization in AKC can induce TLR2-mediated cytokine and chemokine production that can exacerbate the inflammatory response [11, 26].

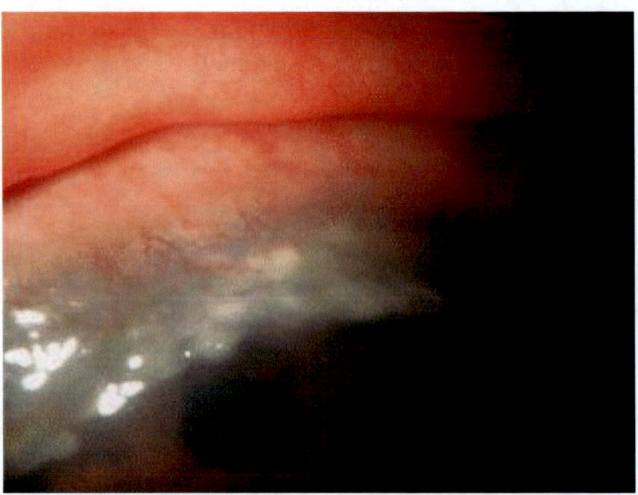

Figure 1. Corneal complications in AKC.

Conjunctival involvement in AKC include papillary hypertrophy of the tarsal conjunctiva, hyperemia predominantly affecting the inferior forniceal and palpebral conjunctiva, gelatinous perilimbal hyperplasia, cicatrizing conjunctivitis with subepithelial fibrosis and symblepharon, and limbal hyperemia [3, 9, 25]. It is of note that not all patients with AKC present with proliferative lesions such as giant papillae and limbal lesions [19].

The ocular inflammatory process and release of allergic mediators onto the ocular surface and tear film is likely to be responsible for the corneal complications (Figure 1). The corneal involvement in AKC includes persistent epithelial defects, macroerosions, filamentary keratitis, corneal ulceration, plaque formation, sectoral thinning, peripheral micropannus and corneal neovascularization, pseudogerontoxon and lipid infiltration [3, 10-12, 25].

Limbal scarring, Horner-Trantas dots and cataracts do occur in AKC [3, 27]. The crystalline lens opacification in AKC usually occurs in the anterior portion of the lens and may progress rapidly to complete opacification [11].

Diagnosis

The diagnosis of AKC is based on typical clinical signs and symptoms of the disease. In difficult cases, conjunctival or tear cytological studies can be useful in identifying the inflammatory infiltrate in the conjunctiva. Skin prick testing or RAST test can be used to confirm the diagnosis of allergy [4]. Although individuals with AKC have high total serum IgE, approximately 45% of patients with AKC are skin test or RAST negative to common allergens [7, 13]. Although IgE antibodies to common allergens are not detectable in all cases of AKC, eosinophils have been found to be present in the tears and conjunctival scrapings of both the skin test/RAST-positive and negative-forms of AKC [13]. It is of note that there have been cases of patients diagnosed with AKC as the sole manifestation of their atopy. However, these patients had a long-standing history of chronic conjunctivitis with bilateral pannus formation [11]. The perennial nature of the disease distinguishes it from allergic conjunctivitis and vernal keratoconjunctivitis, which usually have a seasonal pattern. Furthermore, AKC tends to have lower lid involvement and to begin in the late teens whereas VKC is characterized by superior tarsal conjunctival papillary hypertrophy and tends to affect mostly children and young adult males [10]. AKC must be considered in the differential diagnosis of chronic cicatrizing conjunctivitis and/or symblepharon [25].

Management

The primary goal in the management of AKC is to prevent recurrences by eliminating or avoiding the trigger factors [5]. Additionally, therapy involves controlling the ocular inflammation, preventing damage to the ocular surface and periocular tissue, and preserving vision [10, 25, 28]. Educating the patient on the degree of disease activity and the severity of the ocular surface inflammation, as well as possible identification of trigger factors is a very important aspect of managing atopic keratoconjunctivitis [12]. Patients should be advised not to rub their eyes as this may help alleviate the itching due to mechanical degranulation of the mast cells [10].

AKC is a chronic ocular allergic disease that requires management with anti-inflammatory and anti-allergic pharmaceutical agents, supportive therapy, prophylactic antibiotics, and other non-pharmacologic management strategies.

The supportive therapy of AKC includes avoiding the trigger factors, applying cool compress, and administering preservative-free ocular lubricants. Cool compresses and preservative-free ocular lubricants provide symptomatic relief when there is intense ocular itching and burning due to tear film insufficiency. It has been reported that ocular lubrication dilutes and/or flush away the allergens and inflammatory mediators on the ocular surface [12].

Patients with the mild to moderate form of AKC may benefit from the use of supportive therapy as an adjunct to conventional therapy with topical anti-allergic pharmacologic therapy, topical anti-inflammatory and oral antihistamine. Severe cases of AKC associated with corneal compromise require topical steroids and prophylactic antibiotics [29]. In the absence of corneal compromise, prophylactic antibiotics may not be necessary. It is worth mentioning that patients who present with flare up of their condition no matter how mild, may need a pulsed topical steroidal therapy [12, 30]. Most cases of AKC will require a topical steroid to control the inflammatory process, since T-lymphocytes and eosinophils play a major role in the immunopathogenesis of the condition [31]. Corticosteroid should be used with caution in patients with AKC because of the risk of complications such as infection, cataract, corneal melting, and steroid-induced iatrogenic glaucoma [10]. The chronic blepharitis and meibomianitis associated with AKC requires regular eyelid hygiene, warm compress and long-term therapy with systemic antibiotics such as doxycycline that are capable of inhibiting the action of lipase, an enzyme that converts glandular lipids into free fatty acid. The primary objective of this treatment modality is to improve the overall eyelid health and the quality of the tear film [29, 30, 32, 33].

When AKC is refractory to conventional anti-allergic and anti-inflammatory therapy, the clinician is advised to consider immunosuppressant therapy [34]. Topical immunomodulators such as cyclosporine can be used as a substitute for patients with steroid-dependent AKC. In steroid-dependent AKC, the clinician may consider using topical cyclosporine as a substitute with the intention of weaning the patient off steroid dependency [12]. It has been demonstrated that topical cyclosporine 2% is a safe and effective steroid-sparing therapeutic agent for AKC. The therapeutic benefits of topical cyclosporine has been demonstrated in patients with meibomian gland metaplasia and eyelid telangiectasia, a condition that is usually seen in patients with AKC [17]. Kurt Spiteri and associates demonstrated that systemic cyclosporine is efficacious and safe in treating AKC that is resistant to conventional therapy [1]. Nivenus and colleagues demonstrated that tacrolimus had potential to serve as an alternative to topical steroidal therapy for eczematous eyelid in AKC patients. They also suggested that patients should avoid ultraviolet exposure during treatment with tacrolimus [6]. It has also been reported that tacrolimus could inhibit release of mediators from mast cells [35], as well as bind to steroid receptors on the cell surface and decrease intracellular adhesion and expression of E-selectin in vascular endothelium [36]. Although García and colleagues [36] demonstrated that the topical application of tacrolimus 0.03% dermatologic ointment into the lower fornix could potentially constitute an alternative treatment in AKC that is refractory to conventional treatment, a randomized clinical trial is necessary to determinate the effectiveness of this modality of topical immunosuppressive therapy.

Concurrent use of oral antihistamines may be necessary to reduce and control the intense itching associated with this condition [29]. The eczema and periocular skin inflammation will respond to topical corticosteroid cream or tacrolimus, a non-steroidal alternative with superior efficacy and good safety profile. Prophylactic antibiotics could be considered as an essential adjunctive therapeutic strategy when therapeutic bandage contact lens are used to manage corneal complications associated with AKC [37]. Patients with severe AKC who present with compromised vision due to corneal scar formation, vascularization or corneal ulceration with perforation may benefit from corneal surgical intervention [10, 12].

The effective management of AKC necessitates a multidisciplinary approach-involving dermatologist, allergist, eye care professional and general medical practitioner. This becomes inevitable when the itching and inflammation extends beyond the ocular and periocular tissue [10, 11].

Complications and Prognosis

AKC, a chronic and potentially blinding immune-mediated ocular surface inflammatory disease, if left untreated, ocular surface complications can progress to conjunctival scarring with subepithelial fibrosis, decreased tear production, lid margin keratinization and malposition, fornix foreshortening, symblepharon, corneal neovascularization and corneal ulceration [2, 21, 28]. Patients with AKC are predisposed to complications secondary to microbial infection of the eyelids, conjunctiva and cornea [9]. The corneal complications seen in AKC are usually associated with tissue thinning of the cornea with consequential induction of refractive changes [12]. Consistent with these observations, reported ocular complications include keratoconus and cataract. Retinal detachment, ocular herpes simplex and general keratitis have also been reported [21, 25]. The key to stopping progressive cicatrization and eventual blinding keratopathy is long-term control of the conjunctival inflammation [16]. AKC, unlike VKC, does not share the characteristic of spontaneous resolution [3]. Thus, without prompt and persistent management, it will progress to potentially sight-threatening sequelae.

References

[1]   Cornish, K.S., M.E. Gregory, and K. Ramaesh, Systemic cyclosporin A in severe atopic keratoconjunctivitis. *Eur J Ophthalmol,* 2010. 20(5): p. 844-51.

[2]   Uchio, E., et al., Demographic aspects of allergic ocular diseases and evaluation of new criteria for clinical assessment of ocular allergy. *Graefes Arch Clin Exp Ophthalmol,* 2008. 246(2): p. 291-6.

[3]   Tuft, S.J., et al., Clinical features of atopic keratoconjunctivitis. *Ophthalmology,* 1991. 98(2): p. 150-8.

[4]   Manzouri, B., et al., Pharmacotherapy of allergic eye disease. *Expert Opin Pharmacother, 2006.* 7(9): p. 1191-200.

[5]   Leonardi, A., L. Motterle, and M. Bortolotti, Allergy and the eye. *Clin Exp Immunol,* 2008. 153 Suppl 1: p. 17-21.

[6]   Nivenius, E., et al., Tacrolimus ointment vs steroid ointment for eyelid dermatitis in patients with atopic keratoconjunctivitis. *Eye,* 2007. 21(7): p. 968-75.

[7] Leonardi, A., C. De Dominicis, and L. Motterle, Immunopathogenesis of ocular allergy: a schematic approach to different clinical entities. *Curr Opin Allergy Clin Immunol,* 2007. 7(5): p. 429-35.

[8] Ozcan, A., T. Ersoz, and E. Dulger, Management of severe allergic conjunctivitis with topical cyclosporin a 0.05% eyedrops. *Cornea,* 2007. 26(9): p. 1035-8.

[9] Calonge, M. and J.M. Herreras, Clinical grading of atopic keratoconjunctivitis. *Curr Opin Allergy Clin Immunol,* 2007. 7(5): p. 442-5.

[10] Casey, R. and M.B. Abelson, Atopic keratoconjunctivitis. *Int Ophthalmol Clin,* 1997. 37(2): p. 111-7.

[11] Bielory, B. and L. Bielory, Atopic dermatitis and keratoconjunctivitis. *Immunol Allergy Clin North Am,* 2010. 30(3): p. 323-36.

[12] Zhan, H., et al., Clinical and immunological features of atopic keratoconjunctivitis. *Int Ophthalmol Clin,* 2003. 43(1): p. 59-71.

[13] Bonini, S., Atopic keratoconjunctivitis. *Allergy,* 2004. 59 Suppl 78: p. 71-3.

[14] Butrus, S. and R. Portela, Ocular allergy: diagnosis and treatment. *Ophthalmol Clin North Am,* 2005. 18(4): p. 485-92, v.

[15] Nishida, T.T., A.W., Specific Aqueous Humour Factors induce Activation of Regulatory T cells. *Investigative Ophthalmology and Visual Science.,* 1999. 40(10): p. 2268-2274.

[16] Foster, C., B. Rice, and J. Dutt, Immunopathology of atopic keratoconjunctivitis. *Ophthalmology,* 1991. 98(8): p. 1190-6.

[17] Donnenfeld, E. and S.C. Pflugfelder, Topical ophthalmic cyclosporine: pharmacology and clinical uses. *Surv Ophthalmol,* 2009. 54(3): p. 321-38.

[18] Wakamatsu, T., et al., Evaluation of conjunctival inflammatory status by confocal scanning laser microscopy and conjunctival brush cytology in patients with atopic keratoconjunctivitis (AKC). *Mol Vis,* 2009. 15: p. 1611-9.

[19] Takamura, E., et al., Japanese guideline for allergic conjunctival diseases. *Allergol Int,* 2011. 60(2): p. 191-203.

[20] Dogru, M., et al., Alterations of the ocular surface epithelial MUC16 and goblet cell MUC5AC in patients with atopic keratoconjunctivitis. *Allergy,* 2008. 63(10): p. 1324-34.

[21] Anzaar, F., et al., Use of systemic T-lymphocyte signal transduction inhibitors in the treatment of atopic keratoconjunctivitis. *Cornea,* 2008. 27(8): p. 884-8.

[22] Wakamatsu, T.H., et al., Evaluation of lipid oxidative stress status and inflammation in atopic ocular surface disease. *Mol Vis,* 2010. 16: p. 2465-75.

[23] Nakamura, T., et al., Changes in conjunctival clusterin expression in severe ocular surface disease. *Invest Ophthalmol Vis Sci,* 2002. 43(6): p. 1702-7.

[24] Li, S., et al., Molecular mechanism of proinflammatory cytokine-mediated squamous metaplasia in human corneal epithelial cells. *Invest Ophthalmol Vis Sci,* 2010. 51(5): p. 2466-75.

[25] Foster, C.S. and M. Calonge, Atopic keratoconjunctivitis. *Ophthalmology, 1990.* 97(8): p. 992-1000.

[26] Redfern, R.L. and A.M. McDermott, Toll-like receptors in ocular surface disease. *Exp Eye Res,* 2010. 90(6): p. 679-87.

[27] Friedlaender, M.H., Ocular allergy. *Curr Opin Allergy Clin Immunol,* 2011. 11(5): p. 477-82.

[28] Margolis, R., V. Thakrar, and V. Perez, Role of rigid gas-permeable scleral contact lenses in the management of advanced atopic keratoconjunctivitis. *Cornea,* 2007. 26(9): p. 1032-4.

[29] Berdy, G.J., Atopic keratoconjunctivitis (AKC). *Acta Ophthalmol Scand Suppl,* 1999(228): p. 7-9.

[30] Dinowitz, M., R. Rescigno, and L. Bielory, Ocular allergic diseases: differential diagnosis, examination techniques, and testing. *Clin Allergy Immunol,* 2000. 15: p. 127-50.

[31] Leonardi, A. and A.G. Secchi, Vernal keratoconjunctivitis. *Int Ophthalmol Clin,* 2003. 43(1): p. 41-58.

[32] McGill, J.I., et al., Allergic eye disease mechanisms. *Br J Ophthalmol,* 1998. 82(10): p. 1203-14.

[33] Buckley, R.J., Allergic eye disease--a clinical challenge. *Clin Exp Allergy,* 1998. 28 Suppl 6: p. 39-43.

[34] Stumpf, T., et al., Systemic tacrolimus in the treatment of severe atopic keratoconjunctivitis. *Cornea,* 2006. 25(10): p. 1147-9.

[35] Matsuda, A., et al., Basophils in the giant papillae of chronic allergic keratoconjunctivitis. *Br J Ophthalmol,* 2010. 94(4): p. 513-8.

[36] Garcia, D.P., et al., Topical tacrolimus ointment for treatment of intractable atopic keratoconjunctivitis: a case report and review of the literature. *Cornea,* 2011. 30(4): p. 462-5.

[37] Lemp, M.A. and L. Bielory, Contact lenses and associated anterior segment disorders: dry eye disease, blepharitis, and allergy. *Immunol Allergy Clin North Am,* 2008. 28(1): p. 105-17, vi-vii.

Chapter 9

Giant Papillary Conjunctivitis

Giant Papillary conjunctivitis (GPC) is not strictly an allergic disease, but an inflammatory condition characterized by papillary hypertrophy on the superior tarsal conjunctiva in the absence of significant corneal involvement [1, 2]. It may result from persistent mechanical ocular surface irritation or trauma secondary to the blink action, as the tarsal conjunctiva becomes raked by the rough surface of a contact lens, ocular prostheses, exposed sutures after ocular surgery, extruded scleral buckles, filtering blebs, band keratopathy, corneal foreign bodies, elevated corneal deposits, limbal dermoids or cyanoacrylate tissue adhesive [2-6]. It may also occur as a result of hypersensitivity reaction to antigenic material adhering to the contact lens, ocular prostheses, exposed sutures or extruded scleral buckles [5]. This chapter will focus mainly on contact-lens induced GPC.

Contact-lens associated GPC may result from an immune-mediated hypersensitivity response to antigenic deposits on the contact lens surface [7]. The amount of protein deposition on the lens surface is dependent on the lens type, on the water content and the ionic properties of the lens [4]. A poorly fitted contact lens, coated contact lens or contact lens edge may cause tarsal conjunctiva irritation, allowing the antigens on the contact lens to come into contact with the conjunctival mucous surface, stimulating the mucosal immune system. Tears, cracks, and chips in the lenses can cause ocular surface irritation [1, 7]. High oxygen permeable (Dk) silicone hydrogels can cause a generalized and localized form of GPC. The localized form is more common than the generalized form in wearers of high Dk silicone hydrogel contact lenses [8]. Silicone hydrogel lenses with higher modulus factors may induce focal GPC [6].

GPC associated with ocular prosthetics was initially described in 1979 by Srinivasan and colleagues [9]. The papillary reaction associated with ocular prostheses is generalized whereas papillary reaction associated with filtering blebs or exposed sutures is usually localized [8].

GPC may affect both atopic and non-atopic individuals [4]. GPC tends to develop earlier in patients wearing soft hydrogel contact lenses and later in wearers of rigid contact lenses [8]. GPC develops sooner in wearers of soft contact lens than those wearing RGP lenses [3]. Additionally, it has been reported that GPC tends to develop earlier in patients wearing silicone hydrogel materials followed by soft hydrogel contact lenses [6, 8, 10]. It has been shown that patients wearing planned frequent replacement lenses, who replaced their lens every 4 weeks, had a higher incidence of GPC than those who replaced their lenses every 2- 3 weeks [6]. Individuals wearing low and high porosity ionic soft contact lenses may also be prone to developing GPC with increased severity of signs and symptoms as well as a shorter time of onset or development of GPC [11]. It has been reported that GPC patients who wore FDA type III low water ionic contact lens are prone to developing more severe signs and symptoms with a shorter time to onset of GPC than those with FDA type I low water content non-ionic lens. There is no sex or age predilection [3]. It has been demonstrated that patients with GPC may have a history of allergies to environmental allergens or medications [11].

Pathomechanism

The etiopathogenesis of GPC is part immunologic and part mechanical. It has been shown that contact lenses tend to attract proteinaceous deposits on their surface [12]. When the proteinaceous coating in the biofilm on the contact lens surface becomes antigenic it may stimulate the production of tear immunoglobulin IgE and IgG, as well as activate the complement system to generate C3a [6]. C3a and C5a, complement peptide mediators of inflammation, are capable of producing local inflammatory responses by acting on vascular endothelial cells to induce expression of adhesion molecules, as well as activating mast cells to release pro-allergic (histamine) and pro-inflammatory (TNF-α) mediators [13, 14]. Thus, interaction of C3a and IgE with mast cells triggers the release of mediators. The repeated mechanical irritation of the tarsal conjunctiva induced by the coated contact lenses, ocular prostheses, filtering bleb, scleral buckler or poorly fitted contact lens can trigger the release of CXCL8 (IL-8), IL-6 and TNF-α from injured conjunctival epithelial cells [8].

The released CXCL8 attracts neutrophils to the site of conjunctival trauma or irritation. TNF-α triggers the recruitment of immune cells into the site of inflammatory reaction by inducing the expression of adhesion molecules on vascular endothelial cells, as well as enhancing chemokine synthesis by epithelial cells [15]. Thus, the interaction of these recruited inflammatory cells with tear immunoglobulins and complement peptides results in the clinical manifestations of GPC [3, 6, 16]. The presence of locally produced immunoglobulins in the tears of patients with active GPC is suggestive of antigen-induced immune reaction. The presence of CXCL8 on the ocular surface of GPC patients, which is released from injured conjunctival cells, may be suggestive of a mechanical-induced GPC [8].

Histopathological examination of GPC reveals a conjunctiva infiltrated with mast cells, eosinophils, basophils, lymphocytes, and neutrophils [3, 9]. Although histopathologic studies of the conjunctiva of patients with GPC reveals the presence of eosinophils in the conjunctiva, they do not seem to play a major role in GPC immunopathology, since eotaxin and ECP levels are not increased in affected patients. Additionally, it has been reported that eotaxin-mediated eosinophil recruitment and eosinophil activation do not seem to have a major role in the immunopathology of GPC [2].

The histopathologic and laboratory findings in GPC revealed raised levels of tryptase and histamine, a sign indicative of mast cell activation [4]; elevated levels of leukotriene C4 (LTC4) in tears [17]; increased numbers of CD4$^+$T lymphocytes in the conjunctiva [18]; increased levels of IL-3 and IL-4 [19]; significant levels of monocyte chemoattractant protein-1 (MCP-1/CCL2) [8]; increased levels of CCL24, IL-6, IL-6 soluble receptor (IL-6sR), IL-11, and tissue inhibitor of metalloproteinases-2 [2, 8]; significant elevations of CXCL8 in the tears [6, 8]; increased levels of locally produced tear immunoglobulins (IgE and IgG) [8]; and increased levels of C3 and C3 anaphylatoxin (C3a) in tears [8]. Thus, the finding of elevated tear immunoglobulins and inflammatory mediators as seen in VKC, supports the hypothesis that GPC has an immunologic component to its pathogenesis [6].

Clinical Presentation

The normal tarsal conjunctiva has a satin appearance, in which the surface appears smooth and devoid of papillae. It is a pink mucous membrane with

fine vessels radiating perpendicular to the tarsal margin [6]. The symptoms of
GPC, which usually appear before the signs, include contact lens awareness,
excessive lens movement, itching, decreased lens tolerance, and mild blurring
of vision from coatings on the contact lens after a few hours of wear [3, 5, 11].
Donshik and associates [6] proposed a clinical grading to guide clinicians in
the diagnosis and management of GPC. The stages include preclinical, mild,
moderate and severe GPC. The **preclinical stage of giant papillary
conjunctivitis** is characterized by the presence of minimal to mild mucus
discharge, minimal to mild hyperemia of the tarsal conjunctiva, mild coating
of the contact lenses and occasional itching following contact lens removal.
There is no obscuration of the normal conjunctival vascular pattern. The **mild
stage of giant papillary conjunctivitis** is characterized by mild mucus
production with associated itching, increased lens awareness and coating of
the contact lenses. Mild papillary hypertrophy and mild-to-moderate
hyperemia of the tarsal conjunctiva with partial obscurations of the normal
vascular pattern are present. Patients who present with the **moderate stage of
giant papillary conjunctivitis** always complain of itching, increased mucoid
discharge, reduced wearing time due to increased lens awareness and
excessive lens movement noticed particularly upon blinking. Excessive lens
movement results in fluctuating and blurred vision. Slit lamp examination will
reveal moderate hyperemia and moderate papillary hypertrophy of the tarsal
conjunctiva. There will be obscuration of the normal conjunctival vascular
pattern. The apices of the papillae show subconjunctival scarring and fibrosis.
They may also stain with sodium fluorescein. In **severe giant papillary
conjunctivitis**, the patient is completely intolerant to contact lens wear due to
increased mucus production, discomfort upon contact lens insertion and
excessive lens movement. There is eyelid agglutination upon awakening due to
excessive mucus production. There is complete obscuration of the normal
vascular pattern due to marked hyperemia and papillary hypertrophy of the
tarsal conjunctiva (Figure 1). The papillae on the upper tarsal conjunctiva are
large (sometimes 1 mm or larger) with fattened, scarred apices that stain
positively with sodium fluorescein [3, 6]. It should be noted that papillary
reaction in the area along the medial and temporal aspect of the tarsal
conjunctiva and along the superior border of the tarsal conjunctiva is not
considered pathologic [6]. GPC is usually bilateral but may present
unilaterally or asymmetrically [3]. It has been shown that in soft contact lens
wearers the papillae appear first in the zone of the tarsal conjunctiva nearest to
the upper margin of the tarsal plate whereas in RGP wearers the papillae

usually appear in the zone nearest the eyelid margin [3]. Trantas dots and superficial punctate keratitis may appear in GPC [4].

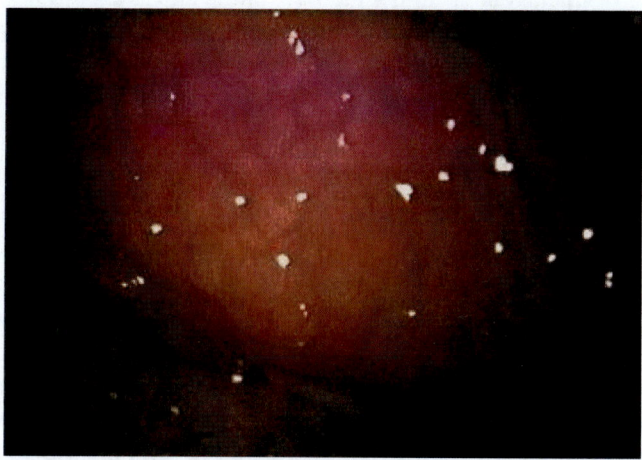

Figure 1. Papillary hypertrophy in GPC (Photograph courtesy of Jeffrey S. Nyman, O.D.).

Diagnosis

The presence of papillae 0.3 mm in diameter or larger on the superior tarsal conjunctiva in association with ocular pruritus induced by immune response to antigens and/or mechanical irritation from contact lenses, ocular prosthesis, or surgical sutures is diagnostic of GPC [4, 20].

The histological appearance of the conjunctiva in VKC and GPC is almost identical. However, the main difference between the two is that the number of eosinophils and basophils is greater in VKC than in GPC [3, 5]. The level of EMBP, which may be responsible for injury to the corneal epithelium, is increased in patients with VKC but not in those with GPC [5]. Although MC_{TC} mast cells are present in both GPC and VKC, MC_T mast cells are present in VKC and absent in GPC [8].

Management

The goal of therapy is to identify the offending agent, reduce the antigenic load and trauma to the conjunctiva, improve contact lens hygiene, modify the contact lens design or material, and modulate the immune hypersensitivity reaction with anti-allergic and/or anti-inflammatory agents [1, 3].

The goal of management in contact-lens induced GPC is to allow patients to recommence contact lens wear as soon as possible with the least obstructive therapeutic intervention. The initial step in managing contact lens-induced GPC is to discontinue contact lens wear until the inflammatory reaction subsides. In certain cases, the papillary reaction may persist even in the absence of the inflammatory response. If the symptoms recur, contact lens wear should be discontinued until patient becomes asymptomatic. At this juncture, it will be beneficial to re-fit the patient with daily disposable contact lens and prescribe an anti-allergic therapeutic agent to reduce ocular hypersensitivity [8]. The modalities that are available to decreasing contact lens coating include improving contact lens cleaning, decreasing the wearing time, and shortening the replacement interval [3, 8]. Enzymatic cleaning of the lenses on a weekly basis to minimize the accumulation of contact lens coating is beneficial and should be considered a vital aspect of contact lens hygiene. If a new contact lens of the same material and design, improved lens hygiene, and regular replacement of lens does not resolve the clinical expression of GPC, the clinician should use a contact lens of different material and design that is more readily tolerated [5]. It has been demonstrated that replacing contact lenses at shorter intervals translated into fewer deposits and decreased the antigenic load as well as the mechanical trauma to the ocular surface [11]. Additionally, regular cleaning and disinfection of the contact lenses as well as frequent replacement of contact lenses is recommended. This modality will reduce the coating on the contact lens surface. Moreover, it has been suggested that patients with a history of allergy may benefit from using a contact lens wear modality that is replaced at 1 day to 2 week intervals [11].

Patients with trace to mild GPC may benefit from switching from conventional contact lens wear to a frequent replacement plan or daily disposable contact lenses. Additionally, daily lens cleaning and disinfection as well as weekly or biweekly enzymatic treatment may be beneficial [6]. Patients with moderate-to severe GPC should discontinue contact lens wear until the inflammatory reaction, corneal staining and apical staining of the tarsal conjunctival papillae has completely resolved. These patients may benefit from daily disposable lenses [3].

Patients with GPC may benefit from either anti-allergic therapy or pulse topical steroidal therapy. The choice of therapy is dependent on the degree of clinical expression. Palliative therapy, modification of contact lens wear, and anti-allergic pharmaceutical therapy may be sufficient to achieve an adequate therapeutic effect in mild to moderate cases of GPC. In managing patients with contact-lens induced GPC, changing the edge design, surface properties, fitting characteristics, replacement cycle and modulus of elasticity of the contact lens could provide enhanced benefits [12]. If these non-pharmacologic management modalities are ineffective, patients may benefit from a topical mast cell stabilizer or mast cell stabilizing/antihistamine combination, using either once or twice-a-day dosing. The dose for these agents can be administered 5-10 minutes prior to contact lens insertion and if a second dose is needed, it can be administered after the lens is removed at the end of day. It is often beneficial to start anti-allergy medication prior to the allergy season, especially in individuals who are known seasonal allergic sufferers. Once-daily dosed anti-allergic ophthalmic agents may be a suitable topical multimodal anti-allergic agent for contact lens wearers who have allergic conjunctivitis [21].

Patients with GPC that do not respond to conventional treatment with topical anti-allergic agents will be able to achieve an adequate therapeutic outcome with short-term use of topical steroid therapy. Patients who have GPC with significant conjunctival papillary hypertrophy or inflammatory component require both a mast cell stabilizer or mast cell stabilizing/antihistamine combination and topical steroid with the intention of tapering the steroid once an adequate clinical response has been achieved [22].

Bartlett and colleagues [1] demonstrated that loteprednol etabonate ophthalmic suspension was effective in reducing the size and severity of papillae associated with GPC. Their study demonstrated the efficacy of loteprednol etabonate ophthalmic suspension in treating papillae. Kymionis and associates [23] were able to successfully use topical tacrolimus 0.03% ointment to treat severe GPC that was refractory to conventional therapy.

Complications and Prognosis

The long-term prognosis of a patient with GPC is generally good; however, approximately 5% of the patients develop ocular complications due to chronic inflammation or treatment side effects. Inadequately managed cases have the potential to relapse and chronic cases require ongoing reevaluation [23]. Although the prognosis is typically good for cases that require non-pharmacologic and pharmacologic intervention, prevention is the best strategy.

References

[1] Bartlett, J.D., et al., Safety and efficacy of loteprednol etabonate for treatment of papillae in contact lens-associated giant papillary conjunctivitis. *Curr Eye Res,* 1993. 12(4): p. 313-21.

[2] Leonardi, A., C. De Dominicis, and L. Motterle, Immunopathogenesis of ocular allergy: a schematic approach to different clinical entities. *Curr Opin Allergy Clin Immunol,* 2007. 7(5): p. 429-35.

[3] Donshik, P.C., Giant papillary conjunctivitis. *Trans Am Ophthalmol Soc,* 1994. 92: p. 687-744.

[4] Katelaris, C.H., Giant papillary conjunctivitis--a review. *Acta Ophthalmol Scand Suppl,* 1999(228): p. 17-20.

[5] Allansmith, M.R. and R.N. Ross, Giant papillary conjunctivitis. *Int Ophthalmol Clin,* 1988. 28(4): p. 309-16.

[6] Donshik, P.C., W.H. Ehlers, and M. Ballow, Giant papillary conjunctivitis. *Immunol Allergy Clin North Am,* 2008. 28(1): p. 83-103, vi.

[7] Suchecki, J.K., P. Donshik, and W.H. Ehlers, Contact lens complications. *Ophthalmol Clin North Am,* 2003. 16(3): p. 471-84.

[8] Elhers, W.H. and P.C. Donshik, Giant papillary conjunctivitis. *Curr Opin Allergy Clin Immunol,* 2008. 8(5): p. 445-9.

[9] Chang, W.J., et al., Conjunctival cytology features of giant papillary conjunctivitis associated with ocular prostheses. *Ophthal Plast Reconstr Surg,* 2005. 21(1): p. 39-45.

[10] Skotnitsky, C.C., et al., Two presentations of contact lens-induced papillary conjunctivitis (CLPC) in hydrogel lens wear: local and general. *Optom Vis Sci,* 2006. 83(1): p. 27-36.

[11] Porazinski, A.D. and P.C. Donshik, Giant papillary conjunctivitis in frequent replacement contact lens wearers: a retrospective study. *CLAO J,* 1999. 25(3): p. 142-7.

[12] Donshik, P.C., Contact lens chemistry and giant papillary conjunctivitis. *Eye Contact Lens,* 2003. 29(1 Suppl): p. S37-9; *discussion* S57-9, S192-4.

[13] Murphy, K.P., Travers, P., Walport, M., The Induced Response of Innate Immunity, in Janeway's Immunobiology. 2012, *Garland Science:* New York. p. 75-125.

[14] Delves, P., et al., Innate Immunity, in Roitt's Essential Immunology. 2011, *Wiley-Blackwell.* p. 3-34.

[15] Irkeç, M. and B. Bozkurt, Epithelial cells in ocular allergy. *Curr Allergy Asthma Rep*, 2003. 3(4): p. 352-7.

[16] Pavesio, C.E. and H.H. Decory, Treatment of ocular inflammatory conditions with loteprednol etabonate. *Br J Ophthalmol*, 2008. 92(4): p. 455-9.

[17] Sengor, T., et al., Tear LTC4 levels in patients with subclinical contact lens related giant papillary conjunctivitis. *CLAO J*, 1995. 21(3): p. 159-62.

[18] Metz, D., et al., Phenotypic characterization of T cells infiltrating the conjunctiva in chronic allergic eye disease. *J Allergy Clin Immunol*, 1996. 98(3): p. 686-96.

[19] Metz, D.P., et al., T-cell cytokines in chronic allergic eye disease. *J Allergy Clin Immunol*, 1997. 100(6 Pt 1): p. 817-24.

[20] Takamura, E., et al., Japanese guideline for allergic conjunctival diseases. *Allergol Int*, 2011. 60(2): p. 191-203.

[21] Chigbu, D.I., The management of allergic eye diseases in primary eye care. *Cont Lens Anterior Eye*, 2009. 32(6): p. 260-72.

[22] Melton, R. and R. Thomas, Clinical Guide to Ophthalmic Drugs. *Review of Optometry*, 2003. 140(6): p. *Supplement:* 33A -39A.

[23] Kymionis, G.D., et al., Tacrolimus ointment 0.03% in the eye for treatment of giant papillary conjunctivitis. *Cornea*, 2008. 27(2): p. 228-9.

Chapter 10

Contact Ocular Allergy

Contact ocular allergy (COA) is a T-lymphocyte hypersensitivity response to haptens that binds to tissue protein to induce an immune response [1]. Contact allergen can react directly with tissue proteins (e.g. nickel) or require activation to enhance their binding to endogenous proteins [2]. Contact allergens can either be a hapten, pre-hapten, or pro-hapten. Pre-hapten is a non-reactive sensitizing molecule that requires air-oxidation to transform into a hapten. It does not require enzymatic-mediated activation. Pro-hapten is a non-reactive sensitizing molecule that requires enzymatic-mediated activation in the skin to transform into a hapten [3, 4]. Hapten-specific Th1/Tc1- and Tc17/Th17-lymphocytes mediates the contact hypersensitivity response that involves the periocular skin, eyelids and ocular surface [5-8]. Additionally, Th22-lymphocytes play a role in the inflammatory skin disorder in COA [9-11]. Allergic contact dermatoconjunctivitis, allergic contact dermatokerato-conjunctivitis, and allergic contact dermatitis are forms of COA. Allergic contact dermatoconjunctivitis, a T-lymphocyte-mediated delayed hyper-sensitivity reaction, is characterized by conjunctivitis with erythematous and pruritic skin lesions in response to contact allergens such as topical ophthalmic pharmaceutical agents or their preservatives [12, 13]. The causative agents include topical pharmaceutical agents such as anesthetics, antibiotics, antivirals, some anti-glaucoma medications; contact lens solutions; and preservatives such as thimerosal or benzalkonium chloride [14]. Allergic contact dermatokeratoconjunctivitis is a T-lymphocyte-mediated delayed hypersensitivity response that involves the cornea, conjunctiva, and periocular skin. The term contact dermatitis (irritant or allergic) applies when there is an inflammatory skin condition characterized by erythematous and pruritic skin lesions following exposure to a foreign substance [15]. Irritant contact dermatitis (ICD), which accounts for almost 80% of contact dermatitis, is a reaction caused by direct injury to the skin cells after contact with a caustic chemical [16, 17]. Thus, ICD is a non-specific inflammatory skin disorder secondary to toxicity of chemicals on the skin cells, which triggers inflammation by activation of the innate immune system [18]. Allergic contact dermatitis (ACD) accounts for 20% of contact dermatitis and it is a delayed hypersensitivity reaction to a foreign substance that encounters the skin, culminating in changes to the skin upon re-exposure [15, 17]. COA is very prevalent in women; such high prevalence could be attributed to their exposure to contact sensitizers, such as nickel. The most common contact sensitizers include nickel, fragrances and preservatives [2]. COA affects individuals of all ages. The skin inflammation in COA is mediated by antigen-specific T-lymphocytes and is associated with skin protein forming an antigen complex that leads to sensitization [15, 18].

The skin of the eyelid is susceptible to allergic reactions because the skin of the eyelid is thinner (thickness of 0.55 mm) than the rest of the face (2.0 mm thick) [7, 19]. It is of note that additional causes of eczematoid periocular skin lesions include atopic dermatitis, secondary eczematous skin lesions in periorbital rosacea, and periorbital psoriasis vulgaris [20].

COA is caused by more than 3000 chemical allergens. Contact dermatitis groups, such as the North America Contact Dermatitis Group, European Contact Dermatitis Group, and the Japanese Contact Dermatitis Group, subdivided the chemicals that cause ACD into categories. Each of these groups have standard series based on regionally specific prevalence data, as well as other batteries that allow for screening by suspect chemical groups (i.e., preservatives, vehicles, and so on) [16]. Almost any substance, depending on its concentration, duration of contact, and the condition of the exposed skin, can provoke an inflammatory skin response. A skin surface with an intact barrier function can deter the penetration of substance, whereas prolonged exposure of the skin to moisture can compromise the barrier function of the skin, allowing access of antigens and irritants into the subepithelial regions of the skin. Patients with atopic dermatitis are very vulnerable to allergens because their skin has an impaired barrier function [7]. The contact-sensitizing agents include metals (gold sodium thiosulfate, nickel sulfate, and so on), ophthalmic medications (aminoglycosides, bacitracin, phenylephrine, glaucoma medications and so on), personal care products (shampoo, fragrances, eye shadow, makeup applicators, d-α Tocopherol acetate, and so on), nail products (cyanoacrylates, Methacrylates, and so on), vehicles and additives (lanolin alcohol and so on), preservatives (quaternium-15, benzalkonium, phenylmercuric acetate, and so on), protein contactants (dust mites, animal dander, and so on), and steroids (tixocortol pivalate, budesonide, and so on) [21].

Pathomechanism

COA is initiated by an innate inflammatory immune response to contact sensitizers that results in priming contact-allergen specific Tc1-, Tc17-, Th1-, and Th17-lymphocytes [22]. The pathomechanism of COA, which occurs because of the activation of CD4$^+$T- or CD8$^+$T-lymphocytes, depends on the pathway by which the antigen is processed. The COA that results from contact with the poison ivy plant is mediated by CD8$^+$T-lymphocyte response to urushiol, a lipid-soluble chemical in the plant. CD4$^+$T-lymphocyte-mediated COA is a type IV delayed hypersensitivity reaction that results from exposures and subsequent sensitization to an environmental contact-sensitizing agent [23].

The immunologic components of the skin include keratinocytes of the epidermis, Langerhans' cells, T-lymphocytes, mast cells in the dermis, and the dermal microvasculature [7]. The pathogenesis of COA occurs in two stages - sensitization to the allergen and elicitation of the inflammatory response upon re-exposure to the specific antigen. It is of note that most environmental allergens are haptens. When the hapten binds to an immunogenic carrier, sensitization occurs, culminating in the production of antigen-specific T-lymphocytes. However, if the hapten does not bind to an immunogenic carrier, an immunologic tolerance will be induced [19]. Contact allergens are xenobiotic chemicals that can cause and contribute to contact allergen-induced skin inflammation, a form of xenoinflammation (inflammation induced by xenobiotic chemicals) [22, 24]. Thus, xenoinflammation is required in the sensitization phase of COA for the activation of contact allergen–loaded DCs [22]. The contact allergens that initiate the sensitization (afferent) phase of COA are usually haptens, which must form covalent bonds with tissue proteins to become fully immunogenic [25]. When contact allergens bind to tissue proteins, they activate keratinocytes to express pro-inflammatory mediators that induce expression of reactive oxygen species (ROS) and cause tissue damage [26]. Keratinocytes also express xenobiotic metabolizing enzymes such as cytochrome P450 subtypes that play a role in transporting contact allergens and activating pro-haptens to become haptens [2, 26]. Contact allergens can interact directly with TLR to induce an innate inflammatory immune response. Some contact allergens have indirect effects on TLR, as they induce ROS that promotes degradation of ECM to yield degraded components such as low molecular weight hyaluronan, a highly proinflammatory fragment that acts as a potent activator of TLR-2 and TLR-4 [2, 6, 22, 24]. Thus, contact allergens can induce the production of DAMP by triggering ROS and hyaluronidase mediated HA degradation. DAMP induced by contact allergens are perceived by innate immune receptors such as TLR-2 and TLR-4 [26, 27]. When a person's skin encounters a hapten for the first time, the hapten binds to tissue or carrier proteins to form a hapten-protein complex that is engulfed and processed by Langerhans cells [17, 25]. When contact allergens interact with innate immune receptors on Langerhans cells, it leads to downregulation of CCR6, which keeps Langerhans cells in the epidermis by interaction with keratinocyte-derived CCL20 and upregulation of CCR7, which binds to the lymph node directing chemokines CCL21 and CCL19 [26]. In the epidermis, the Langerhans cells present the peptide in association with MHC molecules, either class I or II molecules on the Langerhans cells to form an hapten-peptide:MHC class complex. The Langerhans cells travels to regional lymph nodes and present the processed hapten-peptide:MHC class complex to naive T-lymphocytes. This presentation leads to the release of IL-2 by the activated T-lymphocytes. The IL-2 will induce proliferation of the activated T-lymphocytes into effector T-lymphocytes. The effector T-lymphocytes are CD4$^+$T-lymphocytes, if the MHC molecules presenting the antigen are class II, or CD8$^+$T-lymphocytes, if the MHC molecule is class I. The activated CD4$^+$T-lymphocyte differentiate into contact allergen-specific Th1-, Th2-, Th17-, and Th22-lymphocytes, as well as memory Th1-,Th2-, Th17-, and Th22-lymphocytes. The activated CD8$^+$T-lymphocytes differentiate into contact allergen-specific Tc1-, Tc2-, and Tc17-lymphocytes, as well as memory CD8$^+$T-lymphocytes [2, 17, 25, 28-30]. This chapter will focus on the Th-lymphocyte mediated COA.

Upon re-exposure to the same contact-sensitizing agent that initiated the afferent phase, the circulating memory Th-lymphocytes uses their skin-specific homing receptors to enter the skin at the site of allergen exposure [25]. The contact-sensitizing agent penetrates the skin and binds covalently as a hapten to tissue proteins. Langerhans cells takes up the hapten bound to tissue proteins and processes and presents it as a hapten-peptide:MHC class II complex that interacts with TCR of the memory Th-lymphocytes leading to the release of proinflammatory cytokines such as IFN-γ, IL-17, and IL-22. These pro-inflammatory cytokines stimulates the keratinocytes to release cytokines (IL-1 and TNF-α) and chemokines (CXCL8), as well as recruit macrophages and neutrophils to the site of allergic response. The changes induced by these inflammatory mediators leads to T-lymphocyte-mediated inflammatory lesions [23, 25]. This is the elicitation or efferent phase.

Clinical Presentation

The clinical manifestation of COA include itching, conjunctival hyperemia, chemosis, follicular/papillary reaction involving the inferior palpebral conjunctiva and fornices, punctate corneal epithelial erosion, as well as dermatitis of the periocular skin and eyelids (Figure 1) [14]. The acute form of the dermatitis manifests as erythema, edema, vesicles, and bullae, whereas the features of the chronic form includes scaling, fissuring and lichenification of the affected area [16, 19]. The characteristic eczematous appearance of the skin in COA that manifests as oozing and eroded skin is due to rupture of vesicles [25]. It is of note that erythema predominates in the initial stages of COA, but with repeated insult, edema and vesicles may develop followed by clinical expression of the chronic phase depending on the potency and immunicity of the contact sensitizing agent [16]. In the chronic stages of the inflammatory skin condition, the papulovesicular lesions disappear and lichenification and scaling predominates [25].

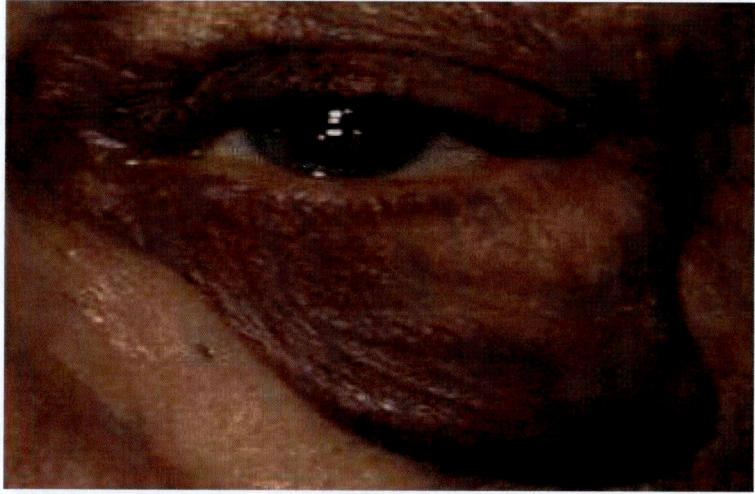

Figure 1. Contact Ocular Allergy (Photograph courtesy of Jeffrey S. Nyman, O.D.).

Diagnosis

Comprehensive history and clinical presentation of contact ocular allergy will aid in diagnosing the condition. Patch testing, the gold standard for identification of a contact allergen, is a useful diagnostic tool for COA. Patch testing should not be performed in a patient with acute or severe presentations of COA, as it increases the risk of obtaining a false-positive reaction and may worsen the patient's dermatitis. Patch test is the test of choice for differentiating allergic contact dermatitis from irritant contact dermatitis [7]. Patch testing is usually indicated when avoidance and empirical pharmacotherapy do not resolve the dermatitis and/or the contact-sensitizing agent is unknown [15]. If patch testing is indicated, the patient should be referred to an immunodermatologist. Adverse effects of patch testing include a severe local reaction, pigment changes, scarring and keloids, infections and potentially anaphylaxis [19].

The differential diagnosis includes ICD, atopic dermatitis, seborrhoeic dermatitis, blepharitis, rosacea, psoriasis, dermatomyositis, and impetigo [19]. Irritant contact dermatitis and atopic dermatitis will be reviewed, as ACD and ICD have similar clinical and histological presentations and the skin lesion in atopic dermatitis could be confused with that due to ACD. However, the onset of atopic dermatitis is in early childhood, whereas COA is uncommon in children younger than 8 years old [25].

ACD is an immune response that occurs in a susceptible individual who has been previously sensitized to a specific contact-sensitizing agent, whereas ICD can occur in any individual if the amount and duration of irritant exposure are sufficient to cause inflammatory skin lesions [17]. Additionally, individuals with ACD complain of pruritus, whereas burning is the usual complaint in individuals with ICD. Furthermore, patch tests are negative in ICD and positive in ACD [18]. In ICD, skin or blood immunology does not reveal activated T-lymphocytes or specific T-lymphocytes respectively [18]. However, in the chronic stages of ICD and ACD, they often present with eczematous plaques with fissuring, hyperpigmentation, hyperkeratosis, and/or lichenification [31].

Atopic dermatitis (AD) is a chronic inflammatory skin disease associated with pruritus and elevated levels of serum IgE. Disorders such as epidermal barrier dysfunction and atopic predisposition are likely to be involved in the pathogenesis of AD [32]. In the acute stages of AD, Th17-lymphocytes secrete IL-17 that induces epithelial cells and keratinocytes to release cytokines and chemokines that induce neutrophilic inflammation, whereas Th2-lymphocytes induce eosinophilic inflammation. In the chronic stages of AD, Th2-lymphocytes induce chronic eosinophilic inflammation, Th1-lymphocytes secrete IFN-γ that induces apoptosis of keratinocytes, and Th22-lymphocytes secrete IL-22 that participates in the tissue damage [11].

Management

The management of patients with contact ocular allergy involves identifying and removing or avoiding the offending contact sensitizing agent; providing symptomatic relief; and treating the inflammation. Such management could employ treatment modalities such as identifying the contact-sensitizing agent, avoidance, good skin care, topical steroidal therapy, topical immunomodulatory therapy, systemic antihistamines, and short-term use of systemic steroids [31]

When the appropriate contact sensitizing agent is identified, the clinician should educate the patient about potential sources of exposure and cross-reacting allergens, as well as recommend appropriate avoidance measures [7, 25], as prevention is the most effective method of reducing the incidence and prevalence of COA [7, 11]. However, if avoidance is unachievable, the clinician should initiate pharmacotherapy aimed at reducing the clinical expression of the disease [16].

Mild or moderate forms of COA usually responds to multimodal anti-allergic agent and topical ophthalmic steroid for treating the ocular surface involvement and palliative therapy with cool compresses and a skin protectant, as well as avoiding the offending contact-sensitizing agent. Because COA is a T-lymphocyte-mediated reaction, topical dermatological steroidal therapy applied twice daily are usually required and could be continued for 2 – 3 weeks [19, 25]. It is advisable to use low potency topical corticosteroid such as hydrocortisone to treat the dermatitis in COA, as high potency topical steroid has the potential to cause significant skin adverse reactions [25]. Topical steroids, the first-line therapeutic modality for COA, have anti-inflammatory, anti-proliferative, immunosuppressive, and vasoconstrictive actions [33], and as such, they can suppress the release of pro-inflammatory cytokines, adhesion molecules, and chemokines [16, 33]. Furthermore, the therapeutic role of topical steroid in the pharmacotherapy of COA includes inhibition of T-lymphocyte activation and leukocyte migration [16]. Steroid ointments are preferred, as they have better penetrability, prolonged contact time, and contain less potentially allergenic preservatives and fragrances [15, 25]. It is of note that prolonged use of topical corticosteroids can lead to skin atrophy, telangiectasia, hypopigmentation, cataracts, and glaucoma [16, 33]. Because side effects of topical steroids diminish as frequency of application decreases, it is preferable to start on twice-a-day application and taper to once daily when the inflammation subsides [34]. It is of note that patients with impaired barrier function who present with COA could develop an allergic response to topical corticosteroid when the degradation product of corticosteroid (corticosteroid-glyoxal) becomes allergenic [35]. This manifests as a COA that is unresponsive to corticosteroids or worsening of the pre-existing condition. The prevalence of corticosteroid induced COA ranges from 0.2 – 5 % depending on the study population [19]. Thus, it is advisable to avoid prescribing non-fluorinated corticosteroids such as hydrocortisone and hydrocortisone-17-butyrate for patients who are at higher risk for developing corticosteroid-induced allergic contact dermatitis [36]

Cool compresses are soothing and anti-pruritic, as well as beneficial in debriding vesicular crusts. Additionally, cool compresses could facilitate the absorption of topical steroid, as well as induce vasoconstriction to reduce skin inflammation in acute COA [15, 16, 25]. Skin protectant, a skin care agent, plays an adjunctive role in the treatment of COA. Skin protectants include emollients (to soften), moisturizers (to add moisture), or barrier cream. Skin protectants provide temporary relief by preventing continued exposure of the skin, as well as moisturizing the dry skin and repairing the defective skin barrier. A moisturizing emollient is beneficial, as it could maintain normal hydration of the outermost layer of the epidermis, decrease the pruritus and reduce the dryness and scaling in COA. The mechanism of action of emollients includes providing a sealant layer on the surface of the skin to reduce water loss and increase hydration of the outermost layer of the epidermis. Petrolatum has good sealant effects and glycerin, a humectant, improves the hydration of the outermost layer of the epidermis [16]. Barrier creams are useful as prophylactic agents to prevent or reduce the risk of COA. It is a skin protective measure that prevents or reduces the penetration and absorption of chemical sensitizing agents into the skin by forming a temporary physical barrier between the skin and contact allergens [16].

Recalcitrant or severe cases of COA that do not respond to conventional therapy may respond to topical immunomodulatory therapy, systemic antihistamine, and short-term use of systemic steroids. Although antihistamines are usually not effective for pruritus associated with COA, it is considered a second line therapeutic agent in the pharmacotherapy of COA, as it could provide some anti-pruritic and soporific (tending to cause sleep) effects [25] . When short-term oral steroids are used for treating COA, the correct dose is 1 mg/kg/day and duration of therapy is usually 2 - 3 weeks. The side effects of systemic corticosteroids include osteoporosis and weight gain, as well as the potential to aggravate peptic ulcer disease, hypertension and diabetes mellitus [36]. Because topical immune modulators, such as tacrolimus have good immunosuppressive effects, it is an effective and safe steroid-sparing option for treating inflammatory skin disorders in COA [16]. Patients who present with COA secondary to topical ophthalmic pharmaceutical agents could be given an alternative pharmaceutical agent if continued therapy is necessary.

Complications and Prognosis

The complications of COA may arise from persistent exposure to the offending allergen, as well as complications from long-term use of steroids. The prognosis is usually good, but severe cases that are refractory to conventional therapy may benefit from using immunomodulatory therapy and oral therapeutics such as oral corticosteroids.

References

[1]   Kari, O. and K.M. Saari, Updates in the treatment of ocular allergies. *J Asthma Allergy,* 2010. 3: p. 149-58.

[2]   Peiser, M., et al., Allergic contact dermatitis: epidemiology, molecular mechanisms, in vitro methods and regulatory aspects. Current knowledge assembled at an international workshop at BfR, Germany. *Cell Mol Life Sci,* 2012. 69(5): p. 763-81.

[3]   Gerberick, G.F., et al., Investigation of peptide reactivity of pro-hapten skin sensitizers using a peroxidase-peroxide oxidation system. *Toxicol Sci, 2009.* 112(1): p. 164-74.

[4]   Gerberick, F., et al., Chemical reactivity measurement and the predicitve identification of skin sensitisers. The report and recommendations of ECVAM Workshop 64. *Altern Lab Anim,* 2008. 36(2): p. 215-42.

[5]   Oboki, K., et al., Th17 and allergy. *Allergol Int,* 2008. 57(2): p. 121-34.

[6]   Schmidt, M. and M. Goebeler, Nickel allergies: paying the Toll for innate immunity. *J Mol Med* (Berl), 2011. 89(10): p. 961-70.

[7]   Beltrani, V.S. and V.P. Beltrani, Contact dermatitis. *Ann Allergy Asthma Immunol*, 1997. 78(2): p. 160-73; quiz 174-6.

[8]   Bielory, L., Differential diagnoses of conjunctivitis for clinical allergist-immunologists. *Ann Allergy Asthma Immunol*, 2007. 98(2): p. 105-14; quiz 114-7, 152.

[9]   Zhang, L., et al., Increased frequencies of Th22 cells as well as Th17 cells in the peripheral blood of patients with ankylosing spondylitis and rheumatoid arthritis. *PLoS One*, 2012. 7(4): p. e31000.

[10]   Annunziato, F. and S. Romagnani, Heterogeneity of human effector CD4+ T cells. *Arthritis Res Ther*, 2009. 11(6): p. 257.

[11]   Souwer, Y., et al., IL-17 and IL-22 in atopic allergic disease. *Curr Opin Immunol*, 2010. 22(6): p. 821-6.

[12]   Manzouri, B., et al., Pharmacotherapy of allergic eye disease. *Expert Opin Pharmacother*, 2006. 7(9): p. 1191-200.

[13]   Blondeau, P.R., J.A. , Allergic reactions to brimonidine in patients treated for glaucoma. *Can J Ophthalmol.*, 2002. 37(1): p. 21-6.

[14]   Schmid, K.L. and L.M. Schmid, Ocular allergy: causes and therapeutic options. *Clin Exp Optom*, 2000. 83(5): p. 257-270.

[15]   Usatine, R.P. and M. Riojas, Diagnosis and management of contact dermatitis. *Am Fam Physician*, 2010. 82(3): p. 249-55.

[16]   Jacob, S.E. and M.P. Castanedo-Tardan, Pharmacotherapy for allergic contact dermatitis. *Expert Opin Pharmacother*, 2007. 8(16): p. 2757-74.

[17]   Nelson, J., C. Mowad, and H. Sun, Allergic Contact Dermatitis and Patch-Testing Education in US Dermatology Residencies in 2010. *Dermatitis*, 2012. 23(2): p. 56-60.

[18]   Nosbaum, A., et al., Allergic and irritant contact dermatitis. *Eur J Dermatol*, 2009. 19(4): p. 325-32.

[19]   Morris, S., et al., Allergic contact dermatitis: a case series and review for the ophthalmologist. *Br J Ophthalmol*, 2011. 95(7): p. 903-8.

[20]   Feser, A. and V. Mahler, Periorbital dermatitis: causes, differential diagnoses and therapy. *J Dtsch Dermatol Ges*, 2010. 8(3): p. 159-66.

[21]   Knopp, E. and K. Watsky, Eyelid dermatitis: contact allergy to 3-(dimethylamino)propylamine. *Dermatitis*, 2008. 19(6): p. 328-33.

[22]   Martin, S.F., et al., Mechanisms of chemical-induced innate immunity in allergic contact dermatitis. *Allergy*, 2011. 66(9): p. 1152-63.

[23]   Murphy, K.P., Travers, P., Walport, M., Allergy and Allergic Diseases, in Janeway's Immunobiology. 2012, *Garland Science:* New York. p. 571-610.

[24] Martin, S.F., Contact dermatitis: from pathomechanisms to immunotoxicology. *Exp Dermatol,* 2012. 21(5): p. 382-9.

[25] Mark, B.J. and R.G. Slavin, Allergic contact dermatitis. *Med Clin North Am,* 2006. 90(1): p. 169-85.

[26] Alase, A. and M. Wittmann, Therapeutic strategies in allergic contact dermatitis. *Recent Pat Inflamm Allergy Drug Discov,* 2012. 6(3): p. 210-21.

[27] Esser, P.R., et al., Contact sensitizers induce skin inflammation via ROS production and hyaluronic acid degradation. *PLoS One,* 2012. 7(7): p. e41340.

[28] Akpek, E.K. and J.D. Gottsch, Immune defense at the ocular surface. *Eye* (Lond), 2003. 17(8): p. 949-56.

[29] Minang, J.T., et al., Nickel-induced IL-10 down-regulates Th1- but not Th2-type cytokine responses to the contact allergen nickel. *Clin Exp Immunol,* 2006. 143(3): p. 494-502.

[30] Murphy, K.P., Travers, P., Walport, M., T Cell-Mediated Immunity, in Janeway's Immunobiology. 2012, *Garland Science:* New York. p. 335-386.

[31] Zeller, S. and E. Warshaw, Allergic contact dermatitis. *Minn Med,* 2004. 87(3): p. 38-42.

[32] Katoh, N., Future perspectives in the treatment of atopic dermatitis. *J Dermatol,* 2009. 36(7): p. 367-76.

[33] Krakowski, A.C., L.F. Eichenfield, and M.A. Dohil, Management of atopic dermatitis in the pediatric population. *Pediatrics,* 2008. 122(4): p. 812-24.

[34] Saeki, H., et al., Guidelines for management of atopic dermatitis. *J Dermatol,* 2009. 36(10): p. 563-77.

[35] Mimesh, S. and M. Pratt, Allergic contact dermatitis from corticosteroids: reproducibility of patch testing and correlation with intradermal testing. *Dermatitis,* 2006. 17(3): p. 137-42.

[36] Nedorost, S.T. and S.R. Stevens, Diagnosis and treatment of allergic skin disorders in the elderly. *Drugs Aging,* 2001. 18(11): p. 827-35.

Index

D

E

F

K

L

M

N

O